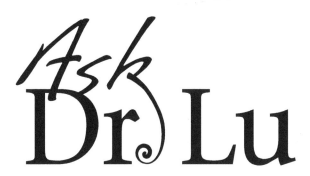

Ask Dr. Lu

Volume 1

True Body-Mind-Spirit Healing
Based on Traditional Chinese Medicine

Nan Lu, OMD

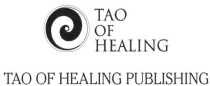

TAO
OF
HEALING

TAO OF HEALING PUBLISHING

ASK DR. LU – VOLUME 1

Copyright © 2011 by Nan Lu, OMD

Calligraphy copyright © 2011 by Nan Lu, OMD

First paperback edition published in 2011
by Tao of Healing Publishing.

For information, contact Tao of Healing Publishing:

Tao of Healing
34 West 27th Street, Suite 1212
New York, NY 10001

www.taoofhealing.com

Library of Congress Cataloging-in-Publication Data
has been applied for:

ISBN No. 978-1-4507-7274-7

Printed in the United States of America.

This work is dedicated to . . .

All the masters who have taught and guided me.

All the students and patients who have inspired me.

*All the individuals who have been part of this book
and helped to bring it into reality.*

*And to those who have dedicated so many hours
to nurturing this material so it can help
others on their healing journey.*

N. L.

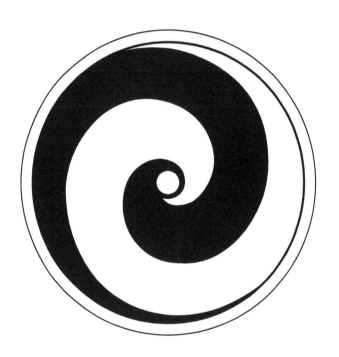

Contents

Introduction xi
    A Note about TCM's Energy Perspective on the Organs xv

On TCM's Body-Mind-Spirit Healing Approach 1
    Listen to Your Body, Not Your Mind 2
    The Body Is a Mirror 3
    The True Purpose of Illness 4
    Our Consciousness Creates Our Reality 7
    Miracles 7

Applying TCM Wisdom 9
    TCM and Its Specialties 9
    Allergies 11
    Anxiety 14
    Birthdays – The Significance of Birthdays 17
    Bladder – Overactive Bladder 19
    Breast Cancer – TCM's Natural Approach 21
    Carpal Tunnel Syndrome 26
    Change – Catch the Movement 27
    Change – Change the Mind 27
    Change – Changing Deep Issues 29
    Children – Bedwetting 31
    Children – Black Sheep of the Family 33
    Colon – Lazy Colon 33
    Computer Overload and Insomnia 35
    Coughs 37
    Dandelion 40
    Emotions Are Life 41
    Fear – Overcoming Fear 43
    Food Allergies 44
    Food – Why Raw Foods Unbalance the Body 45

GERD (Gastroesophageal Reflux Disease) 49
Good and Bad 51
Good – Everything Happens for the Good 53
Good – Truly Understanding What "Good" Means 54
Headaches – Monthly Migraine Headaches 55
Herbs – Why Chinese Herbal Therapy Is Different. 57
High Blood Pressure. 59
Hormone Replacement Therapy (HRT) –
    TCM's Unique View. 62
Illness That Does Not Heal 65
Infertility 68
Jet Lag. 71
Joy – Choose Joy to Get What You Want 75
Menopause – An Energy Gateway for Women 75
Men's Health – Prostate Issues. 77
Men's Health – Sexual Function 79
Menstruation – Sex during Menstruation. 81
Menstruation – Swimming during Menstruation 83
Osteoporosis 85
Outside Reflects the Inside 88
Parasites. 89
Pine Pollen 91
Qigong – Building Health with Qigong. 93
Qigong – Faith Is the Foundation of Qigong 94
Rosacea. 95
Sports Injuries 97
Spring Offers a Special Opportunity 99
Tinnitus (Ringing in the Ears). 101
Toenail Fungus 103
TMJ (Temporomandibular Joint Disorder) 104
Varicose Veins 107
Winter Blues. 110
How to Choose a TCM Practitioner. 111

Appendix. 117

Basic TCM Principles 117
   TCM Principles Reflect Natural Law 117
   The Body Is an Organic Whole 117
   The Body Is Inseparably Linked to
      Nature and the Greater Universe. 118
   Everyone Is Born with a Self-Healing Ability 119
   Prevention Really Is the Best Cure 119

TCM Glossary. 120
   Acupuncture. 120
   The Five Element Theory 121
   Meridians 121
   Qi. 123
   Qigong 124
   Tao 124
   Yin and Yang 125

TCM and Food 126
   TCM Wisdom on What to Eat 126
   TCM Wisdom on How to Eat 127

Resources 128
   Nan Lu, OMD 128
   Tao of Healing Center 129
   Traditional Chinese Medicine World Foundation 129
   Programs of Traditional Chinese
      Medicine World Foundation 131

FIVE ELEMENTS

A Universal Framework

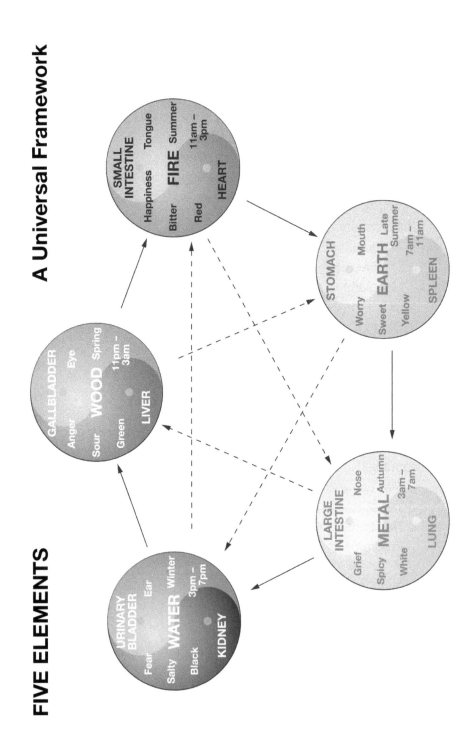

Introduction

People have been asking Dr. Nan Lu questions for over two decades. From the start of his private practice in New York City's Chinatown, in 1990, to his "Questions and Answers" column in *Tao in Your Daily Life*, a newsletter first published in 1995, through "Eastern Outlook," his column in *The Natural Way* magazine, beginning in 1996, and continuing with "Ask Dr. Lu," first published in spring of 2000 in *Traditional Chinese Medicine World*, a ground-breaking newspaper on Chinese medicine, and now in his popular blog, *AskDrLu.com*, since 2008, Dr. Lu has fielded an incredibly diverse range of questions from readers, many of whom have become patients.

The questions arise because people have come to an impasse with their health and are truly seeking an answer to help them restore their vitality and wellness—"to get their life back." Many have not found sufficient or lasting relief from standard Western treatments. Some have gone from doctor to doctor and taken test after test only to be told that nothing is really wrong with them despite the presence of almost debilitating symptoms. At some point along the way desperation usually sets in. If you ask Dr. Lu, based on his practice, many come to him with their questions and search for renewed good health as a last resort: nothing else has worked and no one seems to have any logical answers for them, much less a plan for successful treatment. In the end, most feel they have come to the right person once they meet Dr. Lu.

A widely respected master of traditional Chinese medicine (called "TCM," for short), Nan Lu, OMD, is an expert practitioner of the classical healing arts of China. These include acupuncture, Chinese acupressure *(tui na)*, classical Chinese herbology, Five Element psychology (an ancient Chinese form of working with the mind and emotions based on TCM's Five Element Theory), and Qigong (energy-building postures and movements).

Dr. Lu's unique perspective as a Taoist energy master combined with his vast clinical experience gives him a very special talent: he has a profound knack for getting to the heart of a person's health dilemma—be it physical, emotional, mental or spiritual, or any personal combination of these aspects of being. In TCM it's called finding the root cause of the problem. Dr. Lu is then able to suggest to his patient a way out of the health issue, and he expertly guides them along what is always their own unique healing path.

TCM is the miraculous prism Dr. Lu looks through to help his questioners find the answer they are looking for. Based on unchanging natural law, age-old and time-tested TCM has at its foundation the understanding of energy, or Qi (pronounced *chee*). The TCM viewpoint is that we are energy beings and our bodies are incredible energy systems that support and inform all physiological systems. Qi allows instantaneous communication between every part and system of the body as well as with nature and the greater universe. Discoveries in modern physics have only begun to catch up with the insight of ancient Chinese sages that led to the creation of this extraordinary medical system.

Another fundamental TCM principle is that body, mind and spirit are completely interconnected. TCM's great flexibility and effectiveness as a medical paradigm derives in large part from its body-mind-spirit healing approach. What appears to be solely a physical problem can have its source in emotional imbalance; what presents as emotional upset can sometimes be traced to a spiritual issue; physical problems or trauma can create an excess of emotion. One thing is true, according to TCM: our consciousness is always reflected in our body and our health. In this way we create our own reality. Using this framework, the key to resolving health issues is what Dr. Lu calls the "Universal law of healing": the body has the wisdom and ability to heal itself given natural support.

A TCM doctor is essentially a partner in the healing journey. One of Dr. Lu's gifts is to help the questioner see the ultimate wisdom of turning the question back to the self—to understand the answer from deep within. The trouble is we are trained to seek answers from without. Sometimes we want an answer that will solve our issue right away, and then answer in hand, we hope to get on with our life once again. True healers always take you to the heart of the issue.

From Dr. Lu's perspective any health problem is really a blessing in disguise. "Illness is undiscovered purpose," as he puts it, meaning that hidden within the issue and its accompanying symptoms is a message of vital importance from the depths of our body/soul wisdom that has not been able to penetrate what is frequently the busy barrier of our mind or our daily life. The illness or upset has a purpose, and that purpose is always for good, according to Dr. Lu's deep belief. Openness is required to understand and accept there is indeed a message we need to hear. And faith is needed to pursue and unfold that message and apply its wisdom to create greater wellness in our lives. It's a growth cycle toward a deeper balance, wholeness and harmony. "Without illness there can be no healing, no health," says the master.

People's questions—and the answers to them—are endlessly interesting. Reading this book is like having a private window on the practice of a modern-day TCM healer. Dr. Lu's responses always provoke further study, self-examination (sometimes soul-searching) and growth. One person may ask about something we have pondered many times, and yet in the answer we catch a glimpse of an unknown perspective; another may seek an answer to a question that has never entered our mind, and in the reply we learn something we were looking for all along. Either way, Dr. Lu's insight is enlightening.

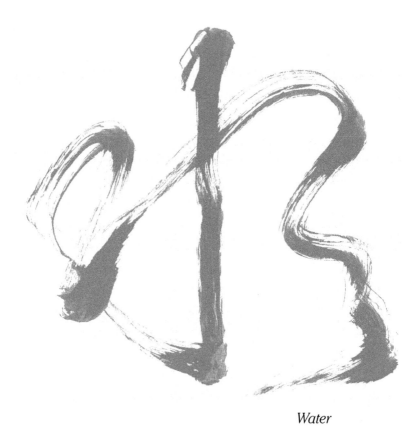

Water

A Note about TCM's Energy Perspective on the Organs

The internal organs are much more than physical structures with sole-ly physiological functions in the TCM view. They are complex systems also involving aspects of the mind, emotions and spirit. Not only does each organ have physiological functions, it has functions at the invis-ible level of vital energy, or Qi.

Each organ, from the TCM perspective, is uniquely related to a body tissue, a sense organ, an emotion, taste, climate and season, among a seemingly endless range of correspondences. These quali-ties are organized by TCM's Five Element Theory within five Univer-sal patterns: Wood, Fire, Earth, Metal and Water. This ancient theory provides TCM practitioners, who know how to apply its deep wisdom in a practical way, with a comprehensive framework to understand, diagnose and treat health issues.

Taking just one organ as an example, according to the Western concept the liver plays a major role in metabolism. Its functions in-clude decomposition of red blood cells, plasma protein synthesis, hor-mone production, the production of bile (which promotes digestion), and detoxification.

The TCM view of the Liver (the capital "L" is purposeful here to distinguish the TCM view from the Western concept of an organ) en-compasses physical qualities like storing blood and aiding in digestion. Yet TCM understands that the Liver also has key functions that Western medicine does not recognize. These include promoting the smooth flow of Qi and blood in the body, as well as the smooth flow of emotions. The Liver has a relationship with the tendons, nails, and the eyes—the qual-ity of Liver function is reflected in the health of these areas of the body. This organ also shares a special energy relationship with its partner or-gan, the Gallbladder, and together they are related to the Wood element.

In *Ask Dr. Lu*, references to the organs with capital letters denote the TCM framework of understanding an organ's function.

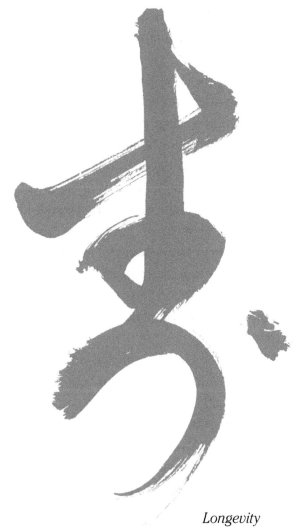

Longevity

The wise man shows us the way to longevity.

When the seasons change, we should mirror these changes.

Challenging nature is futile.

Keeping a peaceful mind and living a simple life
without undue desire allows the energy of the universe
to flow through you.

If your body, mind and spirit become one,
where is the space for illness?

—*Neijing* (475–221 B.C.E.)

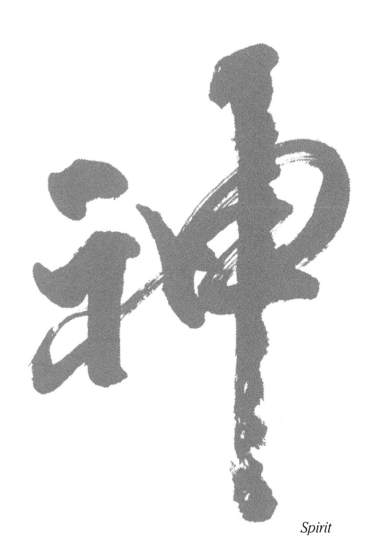

Spirit

On TCM's Body-Mind-Spirit Healing Approach

What is the real purpose of illness? What does true health really mean? Very rarely do we stop and ask ourselves these questions—let alone give enough time to find the answers within. When we find ourselves unwell with a health issue, questions like these might be the last things that come to mind. From the perspective of traditional Chinese medicine (TCM), they are the very place to start a profound healing journey.

In complementary medicine today there's a lot of talk about body-mind-spirit healing. Mostly the body and the mind are addressed; the spiritual purpose of disease is hardly ever explored in a deep and meaningful way. "From the spiritual perspective," Dr. Lu says, "every life has a special purpose and every event in it—including illness—has a positive reason or value." Viewed from this vantage point, illness can become a powerful catalyst for deep inner change.

Essentially it comes down to how we look at what happens to us—what our beliefs about life, health and illness are. Identifying our true beliefs about the role of disease when it enters our life opens up the possibility to discover our own pathways: the one that led to the imbalance and the one that leads to its healing. It creates the enormous sea change of taking what appears to be a negative and turning it into a course correction for the good. Quite literally, a health issue can change your life—for the better—if you allow it to.

Body-mind-spirit is not just a popular concept for TCM, a complete medical system that has been in continuous practice for over two thousand years. At a conscious level we may not be aware of how interconnected the body, mind, emotions and spirit really are. In the last forty years neuroscientists have discovered that at the cellular level our bodies are intricate information networks dynamically uniting body, emotions and mind through the body's own biochemicals. TCM's ancient body-mind-spirit paradigm is based on deep observation and understanding of natural law—how everything works in this reality in terms of both visible and invisible processes. This paradigm has been used by TCM practitioners along with other principles and theories to understand the development of disease and effectively treat it.

It's astonishing that the ancient Chinese were aware of and understood Qi, the vital energy that connects and animates everything in the universe and actually *is* everything in the universe. Thousands of years after their insight, quantum physics demonstrated that everything in this dimension is made of energy, including us. When you break physical matter down, there's nothing solid about it—it's invisible energy. So in essence, we are energy beings. And this energy links body, mind and spirit into an inseparable whole that is connected to nature and the Universal, the source of all and the source of all true healing.

Listen to Your Body, Not Your Mind

I find that my mind constantly strays to negative thoughts. How can I overcome this tendency?

Dr. Lu: The mind serves a purpose. Nobody could live without a mind in the "real" world, in the everyday world. We use our mind to control many things in our life. We send many messages to our bodies. Unfortunately, these messages are often negative and set us up against the self-healing skill that we all are born with. We have to go beyond the mind to have true health.

The outside world distracts the mind. It's bombarded by external messages from all kinds of places, from all the different media. The data coming through our five senses and all the conversations inside our mind cover our true self. In most people's lives today, there is usually little opportunity for silence or little time to escape from continual stimuli.

Each of us is a part of and a reflection of the Universal. We are all under the same law. With the proper tools, we can heal ourselves and rebalance our body-mind-spirit, just as nature can balance itself. We have to look at our beliefs and learn to listen to what our body is saying to us—respecting the body's signs and signals is essential to creating good health. Discovering what we really believe and how it creates our thought patterns and our reality is much more powerful than listening to external sources like media, advertising, and others who can distract us from exploring our inner guidance system.

We should respect our spirit and not abuse it by refusing to acknowledge our powerful self-healing abilities. Train yourself to trust and listen to your body, not your mind. Good health comes from healthy belief systems, emotional balance, and healthy relationships among the organs themselves, as well as harmony between our self and the external environment and the Universal.

The Body Is a Mirror

I know your approach is natural medicine, but if someone has pain all the time, isn't it better in some way to just have surgery to get rid of the pain?

Dr. Lu: One thing is important: If something happens to you, don't say your body has a problem. The body is just a mirror; it's a stage. Your soul, your consciousness, uses the body to send a message, to send an email to you. Unfortunately, you delete this message all the time.

Look at what we do: We have a tumor; so we go to the hospital and have it cut out and taken away. We never see what's really happening. The body then says, "I'm going to send one more message—this time to the shoulder." Then what do we do next? We get a cortisone shot and have no more pain. Yet how can we have no pain? Now the pain says, "You're smart! Let me do more; let me go to the hip." One after the other, the body constantly sends these messages.

If you have physical discomfort, don't make a judgment immediately. Ask it: Behind this pain, behind this discomfort, what is going on in your consciousness? What do you want to say? I always ask my patients, "What is your story?" Everybody has a story. Everybody should win an Oscar! It's perfect. You are the best director; you are the best actor. You are perfect. No one is innocent in the disease world. Everybody is perfect and creates something so unique, but no one understands these things. No one can see how powerful they are. I always tell my patients, "There is another way that you don't have to suffer."

The True Purpose of Illness

What is the true purpose of illness from your perspective?

Dr. Lu: The mind is based on knowledge—from the past and from past experience. The body is built on all the codes of DNA from all your lives because you are not here on Earth for the first time; you have been here for many lifetimes. If we agree that we are a soul, then we have something to talk about. If we agree that we are energy and that energy cannot die or disappear—only transform—then we can say we never die. So therefore, your body and its DNA contain the genetic code to thousands and thousands of "programs." All these programs are based on the soul's decision to choose these two particular parents at the moment of conception.

Once the soul makes the decision to enter this life, you automatically carry two codes: one spiritual, one physical. The body has an agreement with spirit. What is the DNA, or genetic code, that you choose? That's the physical code, but the most important one is the spiritual. Once you choose the spiritual code, the body has to fulfill it; the body is in service of the spirit. Therefore you simultaneously download not only diseases (for instance, diabetes or heart disease) in the genetic code you inherit from your parents, but also the cure for these very illnesses.

So how can you fight the fear that accompanies illness? This knowledge is contained in the spiritual code that is waiting for you to wake up. You have this inside you, too, but unfortunately, you don't see this power inside you—you feel lost. We misinterpret genetics when we say that the body has "screwed up." The body never screws up; the body is always loyal to us; it is always in service of the spirit.

The body does its best to serve you to achieve your goal. But when you go too far, the soul will step in and give you an adjustment, even when this adjustment comes in the form of disease. What we call a big illness or a big accident was just waiting to step in to help you see your soul's purpose. Free will is operating here. Every event has a purpose: Can you see this purpose? If you can see the purpose through the event, then you don't need the event and can skip over it and go on to the next challenge. Once you understand the purpose, you can jump from that level to the next one. If you don't understand the purpose, the event will repeat itself in some form. The health issue or accident merely provides you with the opportunity to experience events that are meant to help you find your soul's true purpose.

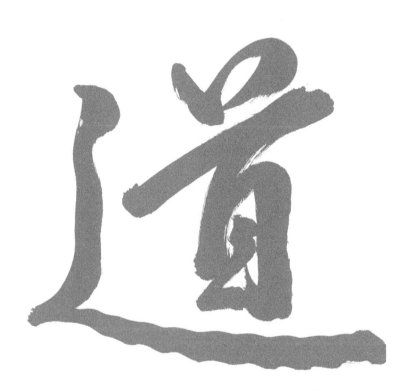

Tao

Our Consciousness Creates Our Reality

Do we really create our own reality?

Dr. Lu: We create our reality—that is true—but based on what? We haven't been trained to see how we create it. Your consciousness creates your true reality. "Be careful what you wish for." Usually this statement is used in relation to negative outcomes. Why be careful of what we wish for? Somewhere, from deep in our consciousness, our wish will come true. That's the process of creating our own reality.

Miracles

Do you believe a miracle is possible when someone is trying to heal from a serious illness?

Dr. Lu: If you focus on disease and illness, you won't see a miracle. If you focus on life, it's much more likely. A miracle is outside of the contract you make when you come to this life; a miracle is outside of time. You just have to meet the requirement and then it happens. What does this mean? You have to *do* something and then the miracle can happen. Three things have to be operating: quality, quantity and belief. The miracle should happen inside the person. We have a miracle every day, but we don't recognize it. There's what you can see and what you can't see. If you see miracles, you associate yourself with good, with luck. All miracles happen on an invisible level first; when it shows, it's a miracle already.

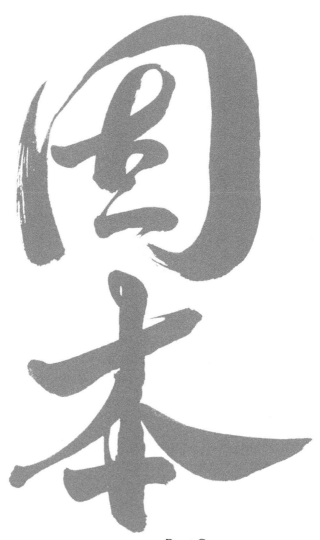

Root Cause

Applying TCM Wisdom

With a foundation of literally thousands of years of clinical experience, the practice of traditional Chinese medicine (TCM) reflects a vast reservoir of knowledge and wisdom. TCM doctors have successfully treated patients with every conceivable type of health condition throughout the ages. Chinese medical discoveries in the areas of blood circulation, circadian rhythms, deficiency diseases (such as beriberi, rickets and scurvy), diabetes, endocrinology, and immunology, among others, predate similar European discoveries, in some cases, by several thousand years. Along the way there developed an incredibly powerful TCM skill set that includes innovative modalities such as acupuncture, Chinese acupressure, Chinese herbal therapy, Five Element psychology, and Qigong. This ancient and advanced system of medicine offers the modern world a healthcare treasure chest that is both profound and profoundly effective.

TCM and Its Specialties

I have read that TCM really excels at treating certain conditions, like chronic pain. Does TCM have other specialties?

Dr. Lu: The essential idea is that TCM can do everything. Pain is one specialty TCM is known for, but TCM treatment goes far beyond just this one specialty. All TCM theories and practices are a reflection of its deep connection to the natural laws of the universe. This is why they have been in use for thousands of years. Modern-day holographic theories reflect TCM's ancient understanding that the microcosm is a part of and reflects the macrocosm, and that the two have to function in harmony with each other. In simple terms this means that TCM recognizes we are a part of nature and are influenced by it. While your body must follow its own internal natural laws as an organic whole, it also must follow Universal law in order to be truly healthy. All the organs have to function in harmony, and yet the body-mind-spirit has to function in harmony with nature, the macrocosm.

Another key point is that TCM is based on a profound understanding of energy, or Qi, the life force that animates all things. Many symptoms can't be explained in Western terms. It's not uncommon for a person to be suffering with many symptoms, sometimes severe, and they just don't show up on Western tests. The TCM understanding of these conditions is that they are a function disorder, a disorder at the level of energy.

TCM always looks beyond symptoms to find the root cause of health conditions. This is why two people can present with what appears to be the same condition and receive very different treatment. TCM understands that symptoms are related to who you are (body type, genetics), how you are (physical condition), when you are (age, time of day and season, timing of symptom), where you are (geographical location)—to everything. Each case and its treatment are so unique. TCM practitioners diagnose health problems and adapt treatment to the specific needs of the person before them. Yet TCM treatment is also based on the knowledge and level of the practitioner. In TCM you can function at the technique level; you can function at the energy level; or you can function at the spirit level. The approach to treatment depends on which level you function on, which level you use.

There are many TCM specialties: sports injuries, women's issues, chronic illness and immune system disorders are among them. But one of TCM's strongest suits is prevention. The *Neijing*, a classic TCM text written about twenty-five hundred years ago, states, "The best doctor promotes prevention, the worst treats the condition." In ancient China, doctors were paid only when they kept their patients well. Imagine that! Good practitioners use TCM to change the person from the inside out. They help their patients identify their problem, help them treat it and show them how to prevent it. It is a healing journey where the person learns ancient knowledge to apply to their daily life, from something as simple as what specific foods to eat to something as complex as understanding how emotions affect health as a whole. The fundamental technique may be small, but it can be used in 360 directions.

Allergies

I'm a woman in my mid-fifties, and in the past few years I've started to get hay fever in the spring. It seems to get worse each year, and I really don't want to take over-the-counter medications. Is there anything TCM can do for this type of health problem?

Dr. Lu: There are many different ways to treat allergies with both Western and Eastern medicine. Some practitioners treat only the symptoms; some treat both the root cause as well as the symptoms. Naturally treating the root cause is best, but this approach also requires the cooperation of the patient.

Western medicine considers an allergy to be an immune system disorder. Its challenge is to identify the substances that cause your body to have allergic reactions. Treatments include desensitization, eliminating or avoiding the offending allergens, and drug therapy with antihistamines, steroids and other medicines.

TCM understands allergies from an energy perspective: the problem involves an energy deficiency. This deficiency can be related to several organs: the Liver, Lung, Stomach or Kidney. The degree to which one (or more) of these organs is deficient in Qi, or internal energy, will manifest in symptoms related to that particular organ.

For example, TCM understands that the eyes are the external gateway of the Liver. A person with a healthy Liver always has healthy

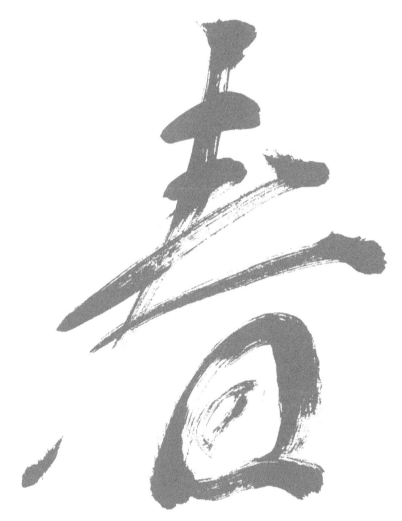

Spring

eyes. If your allergy condition affects mostly your eyes, resulting in itchy, red, or watery eye symptoms, you can be certain that your Liver is not functioning properly. If you're someone with symptoms related to your nose, the gateway of the Lung, and your nose is always running or stuffy, or you have a frequent cough or tightness in the chest, this can indicate a Lung function disorder. Digestive disturbances can point to weak Stomach function.

Because hay fever is a seasonal condition that occurs mostly in spring, sufferers do not connect its origins with the previous season—winter. The Kidney is the organ associated with winter, according to TCM's Five Element Theory. If you exhaust most of your Qi during this season, when everything in nature rests and conserves energy, your body won't have enough Qi left to go through the yearly cyclical energy change when winter turns to spring. Once spring arrives the weakest organ will manifest the most prominent physical symptoms.

TCM is the only medical system with a specialty in prevention, so a good TCM practitioner will help you focus on this important aspect. From a preventive point of view, the best way to treat hay fever is to conserve Kidney Qi in winter. This means making key lifestyle adjustments: going to bed earlier and not being too busy, a state that can cause overtiredness and deplete your Qi.

Classical Chinese herbs as well as Qigong practice or meditation are very powerful healing tools because they increase and balance your internal energy supply. Diet is also an important healing strategy because eating is something you do every day, several times a day. Eating with an eye to including foods with a healing essence can help build your Qi. Add ginger or cinnamon to your diet whenever possible and avoid cold or raw foods, which unbalance Stomach Qi, as much as you can throughout the year. Making these changes and adding these kinds of healing support to your daily life can eventually help strengthen your Kidney Qi and address the root cause of your hay fever.

Anxiety

Lately I feel a great deal of anxiety all the time. How does TCM view anxiety, and can it relieve this condition?

Dr. Lu: TCM sees anxiety as the mind creating the "wrong" thinking. Your mind receives information from the outside and then you "cook" it, based on what you know from your past. You try to analyze what will happen in the future and your limited knowledge and narrowed vision cause you to see something you don't want to see. You create this anxiety because your vision of the future doesn't match your wish. That's the whole idea. There's a difference between how you want to see things and what actually is.

In essence, all religions try to teach you how to see things differently. It is difficult because we cannot understand the new; our understanding is based on the old, the past, what we already know—the old data banks. We always rely on the old data banks, which are limited, to analyze new information. That's the concept of what causes anxiety.

In order to treat anxiety, there are different approaches. One way treats the symptoms; one treats the root cause of the problem. When you treat just the symptoms, the person suffering anxiety doesn't have to change. There's a traditional Chinese saying, "You still walk your old path, constantly buying new shoes!" This means you do something a little different but still retain your old thinking.

Anxiety, itself, is invisible. It is something we create. Each person who has anxiety creates it and has it in a different way. The basic cause is not the same because each person receives information differently; their body processes information differently, and therefore, the response to the information is different and the outcome is different. In one way you can't really treat anxiety because it is of the mind—it's nothing, it's not tangible. Anxiety only shows up in the symptoms, so in a sense we can only treat the symptoms. For instance, high blood pressure is a possible outcome of anxiety, it is not anxiety itself. It's just like bad weather: we cannot treat bad weather; we can only treat the side effects of damage caused by weather, by nature—like the body aches and congested head of a person who has been out in the freezing winter and has come down with a cold. Anxiety is just a concept. What anxiety really is, you cannot say. It's a person's feeling, and this feeling will respond with different physical symptoms in each person.

The first level of TCM treatment is to support the physical body so the body can process the symptoms caused by anxiety. Treatment should make the person stronger, because in order for the body to deal with the problem, you need energy. Making the body strong helps the individual feel calmer, because with anxiety the nervous system is affected.

The Liver processes the flow of energy and emotion in the body. TCM treats the Liver function to allow it to deal with the emotions more smoothly so the emotions and energy can flow freely. According to TCM's Five Element Theory the Kidney is related to the emotion fear. Anxiety always has a component of fear in it. Effective TCM treatment for anxiety strengthens the Kidney function, keeping this emotion in balance. Spleen function is also supported because the Spleen, in terms of the Five Element Theory, is related to overthinking or worry. So by treating these three organs together, the body is strengthened and therefore it can deal more easily with anxiety symptoms. TCM practitioners use acupuncture and herbal therapy to accomplish this.

In terms of treating the root cause of anxiety, the answer rests with the person suffering the anxiety. He or she has to meditate; there has to be a spiritual effort. That's the second level of treatment. To really treat the root cause of the problem the person has to be willing to change from the inside out instead of the outside in. All the treatment up to this point is from the outside in. And treatment from the outside in is never going to treat the root cause of the problem; it has to be

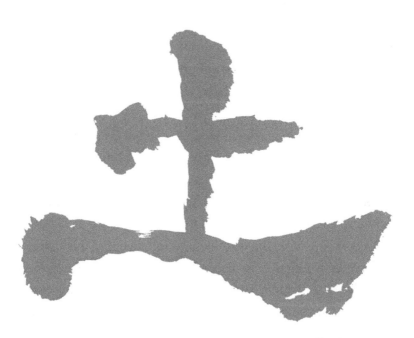

Earth

from the inside out. This means the person has to change the way he or she sees things, and change the reaction to things. That requires meditation. That requires a vision change, a change in perspective, so the individual sees things in a different way: good things are not always good; bad things are not always bad; nothing's all black or white. Unless the person can change in this way, he or she will always suffer anxiety.

By meditating every day, you will grow deeper. You will change your mind; you will calm your mind. You will get closer to your soul. Little by little, you will change from the inside out. This is the only way to treat the root cause of anxiety.

Birthdays – The Significance of Birthdays

How do they celebrate birthdays in China? Do birthdays have the same meaning they do here?

Dr. Lu: Do the Chinese have a birthday cake on their birthdays? Generally speaking, no. Traditionally, no. Right now, in China, yes. Traditionally they give you noodles and eggs: the noodles represent long life and hard boiled eggs represent peace. So the wish is for you to have a peaceful long life! Just be happy on your birthday. Make a wish, do something that you want to do, don't go to work. That's the way it's supposed to be.

I've talked many times about birthdays and celebrating birthdays. What is the purpose? It's for spirit. What is the spirit? It's who you are; it's energy. You have to discover who you are; you have to know who you are. How do you know who you are? Birthdays are one of the best opportunities for you to recognize that on your particular day, many years ago, you came to this Earth—for what? You came for your purpose, for your own destiny, for your own promise. Without this, without nature's promise or the universe's, you cannot exist in this reality. Life is based on this: without promise there's no life. Life is based on the promise of the future: everything will be taken care of—in love.

The year you were born represents the general "contract" to make the elements of who you are. During that year you gathered all the information you would need for this life. Your environment changes based on the year, which means your environment changes and your life builds up your essence, based on what year it is.

The particular month you were born represents action. Why were you born in February and not March? Why was someone else born in October and not November? That has a purpose. The month you were born you had gathered enough energy and information, and during that month you took action. So for birthdays the Chinese usually say the year and the month are more important than the day and time.

We are all stars that come from the universe. And at this time, on your birthday, all the stars should be shining for you! The more you appreciate your own birthday, the more you will appreciate the birthdays of others. It's the same, equal. If you don't celebrate yourself, you can never celebrate others. So I hope you will enjoy your own birthday, appreciate your own birthday and understand the birthday—what its purpose is for you.

Bladder – Overactive Bladder

I am a middle-aged woman, and in the past year I have begun to have a problem with urinary incontinence. My doctor says it is "overactive bladder," and that there are medications that can help my condition, but can TCM treat this condition with only natural methods?

Dr. Lu: The way this problem is looked at in the West is revealed by the name given to the condition: "overactive bladder." On the surface, this condition looks like the bladder is overactive and needs to be restrained. The main symptom is not being able to control the flow of urine. It appears that the bladder is in a state of excess, and that's why it leaks urine. TCM has a different understanding.

From the TCM perspective the bladder may seem to be functioning in a state of excess when a person has this condition, but in reality the bladder is deficient. You can think of this organ as a water gate. A sufficient amount of energy needs to be available to control the opening and closing of this gate. When there is too little energy available to perform this function, the flow of urine can't always be controlled and it leaks out. Usually this happens when there is an infection in the bladder or when a person gets older.

TCM views the cause of this condition as a Kidney function disorder. The Bladder and the Kidney are partner organs. This means that if the Kidney is strong, the Bladder is strong; if the Kidney is weak, you'll have a weak Bladder organ system and the physical bladder will be affected. Why does this problem tend to happen as a person ages? Kidney energy naturally declines as we age. So it's not uncommon to see this problem in a woman your age. Other symptoms frequently experienced with a Kidney function deficiency include back pain, neck pain, heel pain, hair loss and tinnitus (ringing in the ears). All these areas of the body relate to the Kidney. In order to treat this condition you need to increase Kidney function. To treat only the physical bladder is to treat the symptom of the condition; to treat the Kidney is to treat the root cause of the problem.

Also, a problem with Liver function can be related to this condition. The Kidney and Liver have a "mother/child" relationship. The Liver is the "child" of the Kidney, and if it is not functioning well it can drain energy from the Kidney, its "mother."

TCM can successfully treat this problem, but it's a bit difficult because the condition is caused by an energy deficiency. In order to treat an energy deficiency, you have to generate more energy. Generating energy is almost like saving money: saving money is very difficult; spending money is very easy. So in order to really treat this illness you have to generate a lot of energy from the Kidney.

To save energy, lifestyle becomes very important. You have to live in a way that conserves energy. What is the best way to do this? One thing to consider if you have a Kidney energy deficiency is the frequency that you have sex. Kidney energy is lost during sex, so moderation or even taking a break from it for a while is a way to conserve and build Kidney Qi. You should be aware that a very busy lifestyle with excessive stress wastes a lot of energy as well. So does going to bed too late—more energy is required to keep the body's systems active after midnight, a time when the body naturally should be resting. Most people are surprised when I tell them they expend nearly two or three times the amount of energy when staying up very late.

Keep in mind it's very difficult to heal this condition just by resting because the problem has already started. Resting could have prevented the problem, but once it's begun you need to pursue a course of natural treatment. TCM treatment for this problem includes acupuncture, herbal therapy, meditation, and Qigong—this ancient Chinese self-healing energy practice can help you heal; for the long-term solution it's the best medicine. Also, be sure to include foods that support the Kidney in your diet, such as seafood (particularly shellfish), black beans, pine nuts and walnuts.

Breast Cancer – TCM's Natural Approach

What kind of help can TCM give to someone with breast cancer? I was recently diagnosed and would like to use complementary medicine along with the standard treatments my doctor has suggested.

Dr. Lu: TCM can offer women healing support during every stage of breast cancer—and beyond—to help them rebuild and maintain their health. This is possible because TCM has a unique understanding of internal energy, or Qi, and how it impacts the health of the whole person. TCM believes we are all born with a self-healing ability. This ability can grow weak, particularly when a woman has had health issues for a long time, but it is never completely lost. TCM's natural methods of treatment—acupuncture, acupressure, classical herbal therapy, Five Element psychology, Qigong (an ancient Chinese energy practice), and eating for healing—stimulate the body's self-healing program to re-function, helping your body to regain its balance and good health.

Healing is a multidimensional process. This means that your body, mind, spirit and emotions must *all* be addressed in the healing journey for it to be successful and create true health on a deep level, not just temporary relief from symptoms. TCM understands how the mind and the emotions, which are the actions of the mind, play a powerful role in creating wellness or illness, and attracting disease. It also understands the relationship of your fundamental beliefs and state of consciousness to your health. In the deepest sense, all illness is undiscovered purpose—it arises to show you a path to a higher level of health and well-being.

All the many aspects of human health and their interrelationships are mapped out in the principles and theories that form the foundation of TCM. It's important to understand that these principles and theories are *not* the product of scientific or rational thinking. They are based on a perception and deep understanding of natural law. For

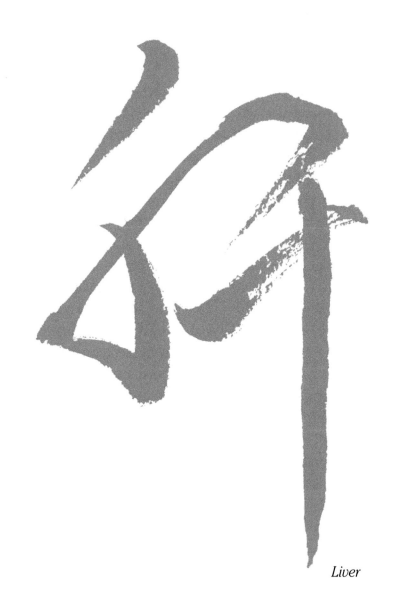

Liver

thousands of years, TCM has used its theories and practices to understand, diagnose and treat health problems.

Most people would be surprised to know that TCM has understood the root cause of breast cancer for at least hundreds of years—that its origins lie in an imbalance of energy. Around 1400 C.E., Dr. Chen, in his work, *Wai Ke Zhang Zong*, discussed this process:

> These [negative] emotions accumulate day by day and cause a Spleen Qi and Stomach Qi deficiency, and Liver Qi stagnation. These conditions cause the body to create a lump. When Qi or energy stagnation accumulates in the meridians over time, a small seed can progress to a cancerous mass. Then the five major organs will spiral out of balance. This problem is called breast cancer.

After you read this passage, it's interesting to know that Western medicine believes breast cancer is present in a woman's body some eight to ten years before it shows physically on tests. From the Chinese medicine perspective this indicates a disturbance or imbalance on the level of energy.

Qi literally means energy, yet it is an energy that encompasses more than just power—it also has intelligence and conveys information. Qi moves the planets and it also gives life to the complex structures and functions in our bodies. Our organs know how to work together because they have energy and can communicate—pass vital information between each other—through the flow of Qi through meridians, invisible energy pathways. From the TCM viewpoint, as long as the body has enough Qi and its organs work in harmony with each other, a person will have good health. Modern physics has demonstrated that everything in this dimension is made of energy. And this energy connects our body, mind and spirit into an inseparable whole that is connected to nature and the Universal, the source of all and the source of all genuine healing.

TCM always looks for the root cause of any health problem while treating presenting symptoms. All physical symptoms are recognized by TCM doctors as distinct signals that an imbalance has occurred somewhere in the body-mind-spirit continuum. Many modern women regularly experience symptoms that they—and their Western physicians—routinely dismiss as "normal." TCM views these as strong indicators of an energy imbalance or organ-function disorder.

The Liver is the number one organ for women. All women's health issues relate either directly or indirectly to this organ's function. The Liver has several key energy functions that especially impact women. First, the Liver is responsible for promoting the free flow of Qi and blood throughout the body. If there is an energy blockage or stagnation related to the Liver or its meridians, very often a woman's menstrual cycle will be affected. This can be reflected in symptoms like PMS, irregular periods, headaches, cramps, and many other problems. TCM sees these symptoms as signs of internal imbalance that, if left unaddressed over a significant period of time, can lead to more serious issues like cysts, growths, masses and tumors—even breast cancer. It's important to know that the Liver also has the energy function of processing emotions and promoting their smooth flow.

According to TCM understanding, breast cancer begins not in the physical body but with imbalances at the spirit and emotional levels. If there is a disconnection from the spirit's special purpose in a woman's life, the intricate relationship between the body-mind-spirit dimensions of her being can become disturbed, negatively impacting her health. Thoughts and emotions are powerful vibrations that can also set the stage for disease. Because body, mind, emotions and spirit are so intimately connected, emotions that are chronically held or intensely experienced can ultimately unbalance overall health. It's natural to have a range of emotions; it's unnatural to hold onto them. The key point is to let them go, let them flow.

Six meridians run through the breast area, and three of them—the Stomach, Liver and Kidney meridians—are where most breast tumors and cancer occur. The meridians work by regulating the body's energy functions. They coordinate the work of your organs and keep your body-mind-spirit in balance. If the flow of Qi becomes blocked in the meridians and stagnates for too long, it can eventually turn into matter. This situation mirrors the concept in physics whereby energy can transform into matter and vice versa (as expressed in Einstein's equation $e = mc^2$), and it accurately describes the formation of breast masses and the manifestation of other breast diseases from the TCM perspective.

The fact that matter can transform back into energy is a very important and positive phenomenon for women with breast issues. It means if masses or other diseases are present in the breast they can again be transformed back into energy, changed from the visible to the invisible. TCM understands that several other factors are also generally present in breast cancer conditions: specifically, a deficiency of Qi and an internal condition of cold. Cancer itself carries a Yin or cold energy.

TCM treatment for breast issues focuses on reestablishing the free flow of energy in the meridians and organs related to the breast, as well as addressing any other imbalances. Because of its focus on prevention, TCM is an effective healthcare strategy for women with breast cancer and other breast health issues because it will help you understand how to maintain your health so that the root causes of these problems are eliminated, therefore helping to prevent their return. This is why TCM really is true prevention—going beyond early detection. As part of the total TCM healing process, you learn how to care for yourself in all aspects of life, from Qigong practice—which helps to break down energy blockages in the meridians and increase your internal energy—to ways to live a more balanced, meaningful lifestyle that reflects your soul's true purpose.

Deep in TCM wisdom is the understanding of Yin and Yang. This

Universal principle offers hope to women with breast cancer because it means that where there is any health issue, its healing solution also exists. When you apply TCM insight and healing practices to your life it creates a lifestyle that promotes true health of body, mind and spirit.

Carpal Tunnel Syndrome

Carpal tunnel pain is making my work as a paralegal very difficult because a great deal of the time I am on the computer. Can TCM help relieve the soreness and pain of this condition so I don't need to have surgery?

Dr. Lu: TCM views carpal tunnel as overuse of the wrist, which causes the tendon to become overstretched. In my experience, it is possible to relieve carpal tunnel pain without surgery. Find a skilled acupuncturist in your area who is experienced in treating this kind of condition. After several sessions your pain should be relieved.

You must also be part of the healing process. You have to take responsibility for your health. Here's one way to help: After being on the computer for several hours, rest your wrist (or both wrists) for ten to fifteen minutes. Then do some soft exercise: Rotate your wrists *very slowly* clockwise and counterclockwise for five minutes several times daily. Gently pull each finger straight out. Another technique to help carpal tunnel issues is to soak your hand up to the wrist in water as hot as possible. Add two cups of vinegar to improve the circulation.

Above all, do not ice your wrists. Even though the cold can help relieve the pain now, applying ice to your wrist (or other areas of the body) can cause long-term problems, especially arthritis. Cold only freezes the sensation of pain; the pain itself is still there. TCM understands that warmth works better at relieving stagnated energy.

According to TCM, wherever there is pain, there is an energy blockage or energy stagnation. Heat increases energy flow and stimulates blood circulation, which ultimately helps to relieve pain. Ginger oil, fennel and pepper oil are warming substances. Gently massage any of these into your wrist and then wrap it with a soft, warm cloth.

Change – Catch the Movement

I really want to change, but sometimes I don't seem to want to change. What can I do in this kind of situation?

Dr. Lu: We all have this kind of problem. When we *do* want to change we don't catch the movement—what we want to change, why we want to change. When you have that feeling, that nothing can stop you, in that moment be aware of your body—how it feels, how it impacts you, and what makes this feeling in you. This will be like an access code in you to regenerate it again, some other time. At that moment, close your eyes and enjoy it: catch the movement and continue.

Change – Change the Mind

Is it possible to do something to reconcile yourself with problems from the past?

Dr. Lu: Whatever bothers you is of your past. In some way "letting go" is high-level "b.s." If something really bothers you, you *will* let it go. If something doesn't help you, you *will* let it go. "Let it go" is a concept that means something is useless. Not being attached to a past event means that you've let it go. If there's so much pain in it, why don't you

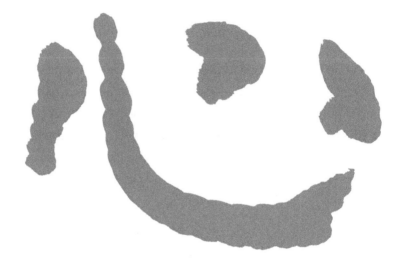

Heart

want to let it go? Who wants to hold onto pain? If you hold onto it, in some way it's useful. Even if someone says, "Here's 10,000 pounds of gold, now climb to the top of the mountain," you will let the gold go at some point because it will kill you to drag it up to the top.

Habits will go 1-2-3 because new things have come to replace those habits. Take an old-style wired/corded wall phone versus a modern wireless phone. Is using the older phone a habit? No! You change phones immediately because the newer one is easier, more convenient. It's not a habit. The same goes for schooling. Every year you learn something new. Your mind wouldn't say, "I don't want new vocabulary, I only want the old." So if something truly bothers you, you'd better look at it. The key thing is to change the mind and your quality of life will be different.

Change – Changing Deep Issues

What is it about our nature that makes change so difficult?

Dr. Lu: We all have a dark corner in our hearts. It's part of our nature; we were either born with this or it has developed through our life experiences. It may even be left over from past lives. This dark corner serves the purpose of defending and protecting ourselves.

In Taoist philosophy, it is called the ego; in Western psychology, it is called our defense mechanism. It's our secret weapon and is very deeply embedded in our personalities. We might not even be conscious of it, but we use it when we feel threatened. It's our power, but it's our enemy also. This is the real enemy—the enemy inside us.

We have to change this deep core issue, this deep innate tendency, or else it becomes natural for us. Remember, when what is unnatural becomes natural, it is very difficult to change. What is unnatural? Something unnatural goes against our deepest nature; it's something

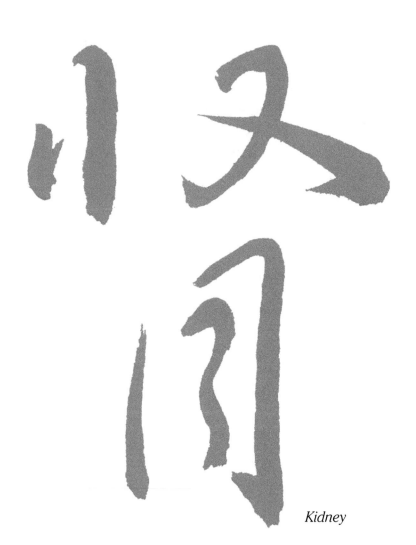

Kidney

that is against natural law. We try to hide this dark corner from everyone; we invest huge amounts of energy protecting this part of who we are, because we see it as our secret weapon. When something goes wrong or people accuse us of something, we pull out our weapon and defend and justify ourselves, and attack the other person.

The interesting thing is that we think that no one can see our secret weapon, but sooner or later everyone sees it. This secret weapon is very well suited to our individual personality. That's why we think it is so easy to hide. We try to hide it, but the Chinese have a saying that mirrors this situation: "It is like using chopsticks to cover your nose!" If we really want to make progress on our spiritual journey, we have to change this aspect of ourselves.

Children – Bedwetting

My son is seven years old and he has begun to wet his bed at night. We've taken him to several doctors, but haven't had good results. I'm wondering if TCM can treat this problem.

Dr. Lu: When looking at this type of problem in children it's important to understand that emotional issues and insecurities can be expressed in physical symptoms. Children are very sensitive. Their young energy is easily influenced by their environment. Stress and tension felt at home or at school can affect them in a very strong way. If there's no way for them to release their emotion, physical symptoms can become the form of expression. It's helpful for parents to be aware of this dynamic.

Looking at the physical aspects of bedwetting, TCM understands and treats it as a Kidney function disorder. The Kidney and the Bladder have a close relationship in TCM—they are partner organs of the Water element. On the surface this problem seems to be about the Bladder, but its root cause is really a Kidney function disorder. In simple terms, the Kidney does not have enough energy to control the Bladder. And particularly when dealing with children's health issues, it's interesting to realize that fear is the emotion associated with the Kidney, the Bladder and the Water element, according to TCM's Five Element Theory.

In terms of treatment there is a classical herbal formula that can help this condition by strengthening the Kidney. Also, moxibustion is very beneficial. Moxibustion is an ancient TCM healing technique that uses a compressed herbal material which is lit and placed close to the body to heat an acupoint or meridian. A TCM practitioner heats the lower back in the Kidney area and also behind the knees. You can rub your son's lower back area and the back of his legs with cinnamon oil. Rub these areas until they are warm and then put a heating pad on the lower back area. Leave it on for as long as possible.

This health problem is considered difficult to treat in the West, but it's fairly easy to treat with TCM. Usually only one or two treatments are necessary to see lasting results. An energy deficiency is much easier to treat in a child because their energy is still strong. To use a car engine as an analogy, there is nothing wrong with the engine—your son's Kidney. It is still perfect; it just needs a tune-up.

Children – Black Sheep of the Family

I don't always feel such a strong connection to my parents. Actually, every other sibling in my family is more like my parents than I am. Sometimes it seems there's always that one child in the family who's different—you hear certain people say, "Oh, I'm the black sheep of the family." Is this because the difference is related to something in some other time?

Dr. Lu: No, it's because of the mind. These children are definitely different. Because they are different, in this society, because of the mind they are treated differently. So they feel separate. It's not their inside connection that makes them feel separate; it's the mind that makes them feel separate. If they really could see this, many things would be fixed, and they wouldn't say those things.

Inside there is always a strong connection to our parents. We chose them! They represent the best environment—the perfect "soil"—for our soul's purpose to take root in this life. We are part of them and they are part of us. Think about it: Is it really possible not to be connected to someone who is so deeply a part of who you are?

Colon – Lazy Colon

Years ago I was advised to take a daily fiber supplement for what my doctor calls "lazy colon." I have followed this suggestion but there has been no improvement in relieving my constipation. Do you have any advice about how I might deal more effectively with this problem?

Dr. Lu: From the Chinese medicine point of view, a condition related to an organ is often not a problem with the organ itself. Chinese medicine looks at the human body as an organic whole. Often, organs have relationship problems with other organs. And relationship problems can cause what TCM calls "function disorders." This is a problem with an organ's energy function.

The colon (the Large Intestine in TCM) and the Lung have a partner relationship. If the Lung doesn't function well, it can cause a Large Intestine energy function disorder, and then a person might experience constipation.

However, when we look at the bigger point of view, at all of the human body's energy circulation, we see that constipation is also a circulation problem. Something doesn't flow freely; something is stuck. In Chinese medicine, we see all circulation problems as related to a Liver function disorder. The Liver is responsible for "flow" in the body. What can cause Liver function disorders in today's society? Stress. Both physical and emotional stress can cause a Liver function disorder. There's something you just cannot let go. Particularly from the emotional and psychological perspective, you will see that there's something that you cannot let go. This stagnation could then show up in the physical body as constipation.

Focusing directly on the colon by taking over-the-counter constipation products might help temporarily—on a superficial level—but doesn't necessarily fix the problem of flow at the deeper level. I would suggest dealing with the Liver function first. This way, you deal with the main problem first. If your Liver is flowing freely, generally speaking, you will not have a problem. Once you strengthen the Liver function, then you can really see whether the colon itself is the problem or the Lung function is causing the problem.

I'd suggest working with a TCM practitioner to create a program to strengthen your Liver function. This could include acupuncture, Chinese herbs and Qigong, as well as techniques for helping you learn to let go of whatever is stuck emotionally. While you're taking care of your Liver function, I'd also suggest taking some honey to naturally support your colon.

Remember, constipation—like all physical symptoms—is a sign from your body. It is letting you know that things aren't flowing freely, and that you need to pay attention to flow in your life overall.

Computer Overload and Insomnia

About two months ago at work I was assigned a huge project and since then I've been working long hours in front of the computer. I can't seem to fall asleep at night, even though I feel really tired. What can I do?

Dr. Lu: A core belief of TCM is that all living systems have an innate ability to harmonize themselves with their environment. One issue facing people in our society that can upset this state of harmony and balance is information overload. Trying to absorb and digest too much information can cause a variety of symptoms, from insomnia, TMJ, and hypertension to literal indigestion. Also, the "soup" of magnetic and electrical fields that we are surrounded with—cell phones, watches, microwaves, and computers—can disrupt our own unique electromagnetic energy fields and the healthy functioning of our bodies. These devices set up electrical fields and vibrations that are different and often incompatible with those of our own body.

A simple way that you can conserve more energy and maintain better balance and harmony is to give your body periodic breaks from electrical devices and too much information. Try leaving your cell phone and watch at home some days. Turn off your computer more frequently. If you must work longer hours staring at the monitor, take more frequent breaks: get up and stretch; take a walk outside, if possible; put a green plant on your desk and every fifteen minutes or so allow your eyes to really look at and absorb the color (the color green is

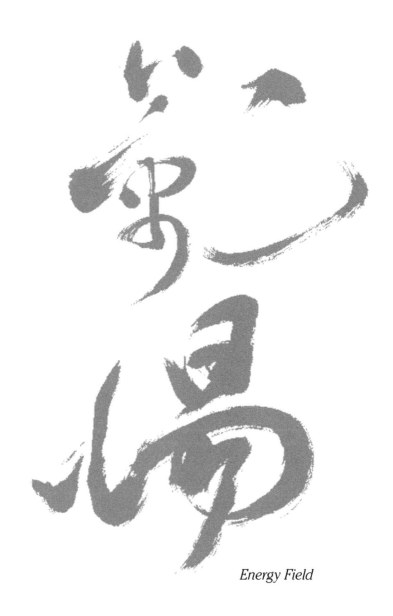

Energy Field

very beneficial for the eyes, according to TCM's Five Element Theory). Go without TV and the newspapers for a few days. Sleep far away from any clocks, radios or cell phones so your body can really rest while you sleep. Most importantly, an energy practice like Qigong or meditation can balance your internal energy and calm your mind. A peaceful heart and mind is the best way to prepare for sleep.

Coughs

Every fall I catch a cold and tend to have a cough throughout the entire winter. This past winter I had three separate treatments of antibiotics, yet my cough still remains. Is there anything TCM uses for stubborn coughs?

Dr. Lu: A cough is one of the most difficult conditions to treat—it is not a simple thing. According to TCM there are many possible causes of a cough. An energy imbalance in each of the organs, not only a problem with the Lung, can lead to a cough. From the TCM point of view, the best doctor does not try to stop the cough, but rather tries to find what has caused the cough and how to release it from your body. Actually, a cough has two faces: on one hand it causes discomfort, and on the other, it has a positive side because it is the body's attempt to release something, such as toxins or energy stagnation.

Most Western treatments view coughs in a negative way and try to stop them immediately. Even some TCM doctors use their medicine in this way to stop the cough instead of allowing it to get out of the body. But if a cough is suppressed or pushed into the body, the illness or imbalance that caused it will also be pushed deeper into the body to remain hidden, and the body will carry this illness or imbalance. Down the road, sooner or later, it will come out as a different condi-

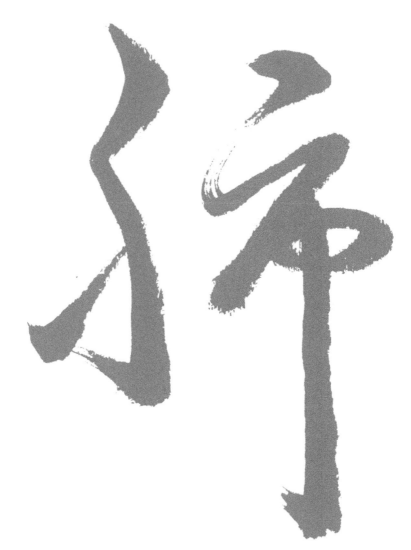

Lung

tion, for example, as a skin condition such as eczema or a rash—any kind of skin condition. Many conditions can have their origin in an untreated cough: asthma, diabetes and even cancer. So it is important to find the cause and not take cough medicine to stop the discomfort of a cough right away.

Because TCM sees a cough as being potentially related to different organs, TCM doctors look at symptoms accompanying a cough in order to understand and diagnose it correctly. Sometimes a person feels some nausea when coughing. A cough can cause rib pain or send you running to the bathroom to urinate. If your cough causes nausea, it may be related to a Stomach problem. If your ribs feel painful when you cough, this can indicate a Liver imbalance. If coughing makes you urinate, your Bladder may be having difficulties.

In your case, because you seem to catch a cold every fall and in TCM the fall is related to the Lung, this organ is most likely vulnerable for you. At this time of year you should take care to avoid stress and conditions that can lead to a cold. According to TCM, the Lung and the Kidney have a close energy relationship. The Kidney, the organ related to the winter season, is the "child" of the Lung, meaning the Lung supports and nourishes the Kidney. So it is possible that your Kidney has an energy deficiency that prevents your body from healing the cough during the winter, and so it is carried over into the spring.

To treat a cough, once its root cause has been found, a TCM doctor uses acupuncture on specific meridians related to the distressed organ or organs. Classical Chinese herbs are also used to address the root cause. Certain foods can help this condition, for instance, a dish of pears cooked with almonds and honey is very beneficial for a cough.

Dandelion

What are dandelions greens used for in TCM? You have suggested that my wife eat them on a regular basis.

Dr. Lu: The dandelion is one of the most profound things nature has created. You can find it around almost the whole world. It's amazing! Certain kinds of plants cannot grow in some places. But the dandelion—America has dandelions, Europe has them, and China does also. That seed starts the whole thing. That seed, that flower . . . the wind blows and they just go! The dandelion doesn't care, it goes with the flow. When the flower is finished, it turns and becomes the seed pod. Then the wind blows and the next generation moves. How good it is! Just look at this and you will understand. You can write a whole poem, a whole story, just about the dandelion, and the nature and essence of it.

TCM uses dandelion greens for many things. Their energy essence, which is cool, travels to the Liver, Stomach and Lung meridians. Dandelion greens are a natural tonic for the digestive system, especially the Liver and Stomach. Because they help relieve the body of internal heat and dampness, TCM practitioners prescribe them for digestive problems that are caused by these internal conditions. Eating dandelion greens can help relieve constipation. Dandelion is a natural antibiotic; it can help heal skin problems and infections. From ancient times TCM practitioners have made a paste by smashing the greens to a pulp. This mixture is then applied to the area affected with an infection or sore. Traditionally it has been used for breast area issues. Dandelion wine is the best for breast cancer prevention.

If you eat dandelions twice a week, they can really do something for your health. Women can gain breast health; men can get skin health. You can eat the whole dandelion: the flowers, leaves (greens) and the root. All of it is from the earth. Cut the flowers and you can have a flower salad—just dandelion flowers. Or you can cut the leaves and sauté them. You'll help build your health from the inside out if you eat dandelions.

Emotions Are Life

I'm a person who has great difficulty controlling my emotions. They get out of hand and get the best of me before I realize what's happening. Are some people just more emotional than others? How does TCM view emotions and are there any effective TCM techniques for controlling our emotions?

Dr. Lu: Emotion is the true feeling of your consciousness. It's all based on how you want to receive information. You then process the information you receive. For example, if you are sad, you gather information to feed the sadness. This emotion resonates with the Lung (sadness is associated with the Lung according to TCM's Five Element Theory). It means you still have a healthy Lung in order to be able to do this.

Emotions are Life; without them you're just a piece of meat! They are positive, not negative. It all depends on how you want to see things. Emotions are a screen; they are a picture of something. If you are angry, acknowledge your anger. No matter what has made you angry, you are absolutely right—from your own angle, from what you see, you have every right to be angry. But don't get stuck there! You have to see why you get angry. Once you know you are angry, you have to go to the next step—change!

With thirty different people, one event would stimulate something different in each person. Some might laugh at what happened; some would get angry. The point is this: You have to change. Otherwise, the emotion will eventually express itself in a symptom. So don't think "negative" emotions are bad. You are alive! You are able to see things. Be true to yourself, and if you are angry, find out why you are angry. Then change the way you see things.

Consider this: Take any object, depending on where you sit in front of that object, you'll see something different. All that really changes is the change of angle. It's simple. A stone is a simple example of how you can look at things from a different angle. From one side the stone may appear smooth and white in color. If you turn it just a little, it may show jagged areas and black lines. Which is the true perception? Both! If you can turn your perception of events and people in this way, you can free up the energy trapped in the emotion. Look at the weather: nature can change on a dime. If you know how to be flexible like nature, things that happen in your life will not be a problem.

How you receive emotions is based on your thoughts. You can change your thoughts. They are a program, just like on TV. It's up to you. What do you want to see? If you don't like the reality you see, you can change the channel! It's up to you. This is a basic principle. There are many specific examples to illustrate this principle. For instance, a woman finds herself filled with anger after waiting over three hours to see her doctor. It just makes her wild with anger. We have to look closely at our emotions and our thoughts. In any given situation where emotion is out of balance, our relationship to that situation is out of balance. Change the relationship to the situation! In the case of the woman mentioned above, she needs to become aware that *she* chose the doctor, and *she* then put herself into that system and all it brings with it. The doctor has to follow the system he or she is part of. If you don't like what the system holds for you, change it! If you change, you won't need that system, so you will go to a different doctor in another system. One day, you may find that you don't even need a doctor.

You have the power to use you emotion wisely. It's your energy. Move this energy to a different level. It's important to realize that you never do something that you don't need. Remember, the universe always provides what you need, not necessarily what you want.

Fear – Overcoming Fear

From the time I was a girl I have experienced periods in my life where I've been overtaken by feelings of intense fear. When I have this fear, it can really shut down my life. I tend to become very self-protective: I don't want to go out and I don't really want to see anyone. Do you have any suggestion for me to understand this better so I can move forward in my life?

Dr. Lu: You should find out exactly what makes you afraid. You are not afraid of everything. Most of the time fear does not exist. You feel fear for what reason? What are you truly afraid of? Try to look deep within yourself and be honest about your own feelings. Without clearing up this kind of fear, you will always limit yourself in your life.

What you call "self-protection" is not really protection. Look deeply at this concept. What are you protecting? What are you afraid to lose? The past allows you to hold onto a certain feeling. You try to hold or protect something that is not real. Ask yourself this question: Is it worth it to hold this image and lose your unlimited possibility for the future? We have to look at what the "profit" is from our "image" issues. You don't really gain anything. Bottom line, you are unhappy, otherwise you would not seek guidance.

There is a positive way to look at this situation. Tell yourself, "It's important to discover who I am." You are going to think about yourself, so why don't you think in a positive way instead of thinking about the bad, the fears, and so on? Remember, no one forces you to think about the bad. You have a choice. If you have a choice, why don't you think about the good? When you think about the good, you feel good. This makes the energy flow. Just saying, "I'm happy," the image in front of you is good. When you say, "I'm stressed," you think of your job or the other things that create stress in your life. Life is for fulfillment of your life commitment, to experience something that will add to your life enjoyment. Not many people train themselves to see or focus on the good. Change to this way of looking at things and associate with the good, and see what happens.

Food Allergies

I have food allergies. How does TCM view this health issue? Is fasting a solution?

Dr. Lu: When your stomach cannot handle food, what's happening? Every food on Earth is useful. Otherwise it would not be here. Food is something natural; it's a part of nature. No food creates allergies. The only issue behind allergies is the thing that makes us unable to process that particular food. So when you have a food allergy, you have to look at the purpose: what the specific food represents in your life. If food creates a problem for you, look deeply and see what it really means in your life.

Looking at food allergies from the perspective of prevention, for example, why do you have a food allergy today when you didn't have one five years ago? Little by little, a particular food has caused you problems until one day, you say, "I can't eat this food, it's bad for me." Practically speaking, it may be useful to avoid this food at that point, but the food itself is not the issue. Avoidance is not prevention. The food has assumed enemy status—something to fear.

In the TCM view, a food allergy can be a signal that an unbalanced relationship exists in your life. The particular food acts as a messenger to point this out. If you go deeper, you might see where this problem exists and rebalance this relationship. Once addressed, true health can return. Is the unbalanced relationship between your body and mind? Is it between you and the environment? Is it between you and your family? You and work? If these relationships are not healed, then you might develop allergies to even more foods until the root cause is fixed. Food has a natural purpose—to nurture and sustain us. Food is not bad.

And remember, the stomach is not just about food; information is also digested. A "disturbed" stomach—an upset stomach—often shows an un-peaceful mind. Fasting means nothing is coming into the body. But it's not just food you need to refrain from every so often, it's also information and emotions that you need to take a break from. The purpose of fasting is to bring your body to a healthy place, a balanced place. Then you can eat whatever you want, and that is freedom when it comes to food and your life.

Food – Why Raw Foods Unbalance the Body

I have heard TCM doctors do not believe it is healthy to eat salads and raw vegetables during the summer. Is this true?

Dr. Lu: What you eat is important because it's something you do every day, several times a day. Therefore your diet can definitely affect your overall health. Chinese medicine believes that anything you do on a daily basis can have a great impact on your health. Good practices, like a balanced diet and meditation, are very powerful because they can actually build your health gradually over time; poor choices can destroy it.

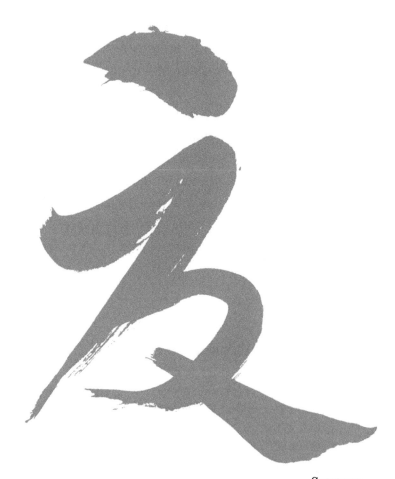

Summer

It's true that TCM suggests you follow the seasons when it comes to what you eat, but unfortunately, eating raw foods during the summer is not what is meant by "following the seasons." Why? Each organ has a natural "preference." This preference is not something someone made up along the way but is natural law—how nature and everything in it works at the energy level. This includes your body!

In TCM, when we talk about energy or the energy essence of particular foods, we move beyond physical qualities like nutritional value, vitamins or calories. In the TCM concept, essence refers to how substances like food and herbs, which are another TCM healing tool, affect the body: which meridians they go to, which organs are impacted, and how the substance affects your body's overall Qi, or internal energy.

The Stomach's nature is to love warmth and dislike cold energies. This means that cold and icy foods and drinks actually go against what is natural for the Stomach and unbalance its function—its energy function; they also unbalance the function of the Spleen, its partner organ. Raw food, which has a cold essence, also goes against the Stomach's natural preference. It's true that raw food has slightly more nutrition than cooked food, but the amount of energy your Stomach has to "spend" to digest raw food more than cancels out that advantage. So continually eating raw foods at any time of the year can have a negative effect on your body because they unbalance the function of the digestive organs.

Your body will eventually show signs that your Stomach function is being affected by eating raw foods with symptoms like gas, bloating, gurgling sounds, burping, stomach distention and pain. Over a long period of time other organs can also be affected because all the organs are interrelated.

What are the right foods to eat in each season? Generally speaking, native or local foods that are available in the season are best. Most

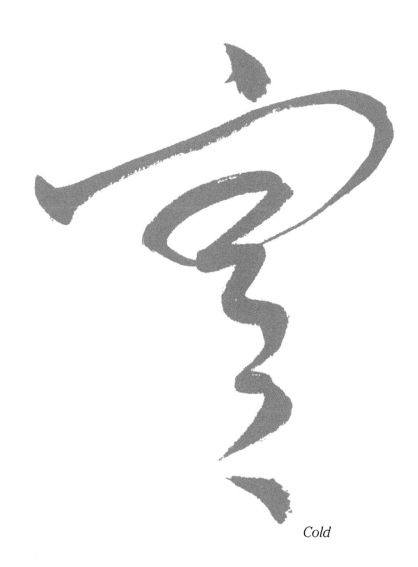

Cold

people don't eat this way anymore because food is shipped from all around the world. The universe never makes a mistake—it always provides the right thing in the right season. TCM's ancient Five Element Theory provides a natural framework to understand which particular foods are most healing to eat in each season. And be sure to cook or lightly steam your vegetables—just a few minutes in boiling water will help your Stomach process them more effectively.

GERD (Gastroesophogeal Reflux Disease)

I'm a 47-year-old man and I've recently been diagnosed with acid reflux. I'm active and eat pretty well, so I'm surprised to have this condition. What does TCM see as the cause of it?

Dr. Lu: I see many patients with this kind of condition. GERD is the Western medical term for the symptoms that result when gastric contents like stomach acid flow back up the esophagus, the canal extending from the pharynx to the stomach. This is a fairly common condition.

Research by the National Institutes of Health (NIH) reveals that more than 60 million people suffer heartburn associated with acid reflux at least once a month, and about 25 million people have this symptom on a daily basis. In most cases, they have sought relief from the symptoms of GERD—heartburn, bloating, regurgitation, burping, sore throat, bad breath, hoarseness, dry cough (especially at night), asthma, and chest discomfort or pain—with over-the-counter medications, sometimes using them over a long period of time. These products cannot eliminate GERD completely because they do not address its root cause.

TCM has been treating this condition for centuries. The first known herbal formula for it was recorded in 210 C.E. From the TCM viewpoint, GERD is caused by a Liver and Stomach function disorder. A "function disorder," in TCM terms, refers to an imbalance at the level of energy. Most often, an excess of emotions, like anger and frustration, and/or too much stress is the underlying root cause of a Liver dysfunction. Part of the Liver's energy function is to regulate or maintain the smooth flow of emotion in the body-mind-spirit. Understanding this concept, it's fairly easy to see how an excess of emotion and stress creates extra "work" for the Liver and can unbalance its health overall.

Usually, poor diet habits are the real source of a Stomach dysfunction. The energy (Qi) of the Stomach is naturally supposed to flow downward in the body. Too much stress can cause it to move upward, causing some of the uncomfortable symptoms of GERD. Though Western medicine refers to this condition as heartburn, in classical Chinese medical literature it has nothing to do with the heart.

Like you, many of my Western patients believe they are eating a healthy, well-balanced diet. However, it's important to understand that the Stomach, as TCM understands its energy requirements, has a natural inclination for warm foods and beverages. This means foods that are cooked or steamed, like soups or steamed vegetables, and drinks like hot tea. Also, foods with a warm energy essence are beneficial for the Stomach. The energy essence of any food is what actually makes it a healing substance for the body. Ginger, cinnamon and fennel have a warm essence. If your diet includes a steady stream of cold food like ice cream and cold salads, or if you constantly drink iced beverages, you are unbalancing the energy of your Stomach. Also, foods with a cold energy essence, such as raw foods or root vegetables, can impair Stomach function. Be aware that too much fried food and dairy products can cause or aggravate GERD. To strengthen your Stomach Qi, make sure you're eating according to TCM principles (see Appendix).

Good and Bad

As a Western person approaching an Eastern system of spirituality, I find some major differences. One is the way Westerners view the world, people and events in black and white, as "good" or "bad." I understand that in the Taoist system there is no good or bad. Can you help me understand this?

Dr. Lu: If you want to challenge yourself in a big way, you have to let go of what you call all the "good" and "bad" experiences. Process them and let them go. You have to accept all of your positive and negative reactions to people, situations and experiences, process your reactions and let them go. You have to see and accept the positive and negative sides of yourself. This involves a big-heartedness and humility. You accept yourself and you accept everything. Take it all in and then let it go, all the while not losing sight of your place in the big picture, your mission and your destiny.

In this life, we have to make judgments of good and bad. At the beginning of the spiritual journey it is natural to think this way. But for those who have been on the path for a while, there should be a change in how you see the world. This understanding of what is good and what is bad should change in certain stages.

The first level is to know what is bad. The second is to know what is good. At the third level, we try to do what we perceive as good and avoid doing what we see as bad. The fourth and highest level is to understand that good and bad are just two different sides of the whole. Then we can accept everything. Good and bad are opposite sides of the same coin and contain the same quantity of energy. When a criminal converts and changes his ways, he has the potential to become as good as he was bad. We come to understand the truth of the Tao: that there is no good or bad. These categories are based on our judgments; they are not real.

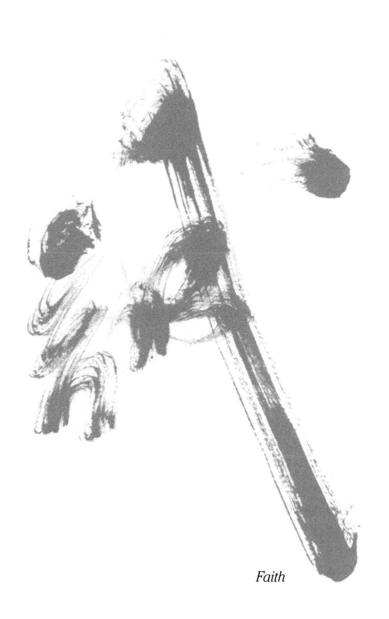

Faith

We all have to accept the level that we are on. If we are on the level of still seeing good and bad, then we should have the passion to do only good. On this level of judgment we suffer because we are neither one hundred percent good, nor one hundred percent bad. A person one hundred percent bad has to follow his destiny also. In so doing, this person causes many people to change. We have to trust what life presents, no matter what it looks like on the outside. The truth lies deep within, deeper than our judgments of good and bad. If you go deep you will find this truth.

Good – Everything Happens for the Good

If we want something for our future, should we imagine it now?

Dr. Lu: Not necessarily, because at your level now you may not imagine what is really yours. You may imagine certain things, but they may never exist in this reality—perhaps only in the dream level. A dream is just a different kind of reality; it still tells you the truth.

We need to change our beliefs. This applies to our belief about our future. We have to believe it will provide the best for us, no matter what. Most people think they have to do more to plan for or control what happens in their future. But a healthy belief to have is this: I will do less for my future and then natural law will operate to give me what is best for me.

You need to accept that everything that happens to you is for the good. To maximize your self-cultivation practice and open up your life you have to change to this belief. The past will not bother you because everything is for good. But you have to believe it in your core. Old clothes are a good example of this: we hang onto them even though they are of no use and we never wear them anymore.

"Trying" to believe everything that happens to you is for good is the hard way to go. Everybody is capable of believing anything! Look at the positive side: Everything happens for a good reason. It's even possible to get bread for free! Why not? Maybe the baker owes you. When you think this way your life will change. If you look at things this way you will see the good and you will experience the good. We want to avoid bad, but we are looking for—expecting—bad, and so we get bad.

This belief—that everything that happens to you is for the good—is a tool for spiritual growth. Maybe one day you go a different way to work and that causes you to miss an accident. The new path is quick; you don't have to pay a toll. Why not try the new path? The old path is still there if this tool doesn't work for you. I'm asking you to open your mind.

Everything happens to you for a reason. The reason is to help you grow and discover who you are. All of fate is perfect. Life is perfect. Believing or seeing that it is perfect makes it easier to go through it.

Good – Truly Understanding What "Good" Means

If you find yourself in a life situation that makes you really tired or even makes you sick sometimes, and you can't leave it right away, how can you deal with it in a positive way? I have heard you say that everything happens to us for the good. Please help me understand how a difficult situation can be good for me.

Dr. Lu: You have to change. You cannot just say, "I believe everything that happens to me is for the good." No! It *is* good, but can you *see* the good? You cannot just lie to yourself saying, "It's good." That's not good! Every day, every night, you work late, you are unhappy . . . it's for good. Your boyfriend gives you a hard time . . . it's for good. It's not for good! You might want to quit your job; you might want to punch your boyfriend's face. How can it be for good? Unless you truly understand what's happening.

What is good? What does this really mean? The good is *you have to change.* It's not just good. Good is how can I change so life situations won't bother me anymore? Your boss will understand you; now, he wants to give you a hard time. You start to think, "Maybe when I change he won't give me a hard time, he will help me." See, that's more positive instead of just saying, "Oh yea, he gives me a hard time instead of helping me." Can you change for your own benefit, for good? Good means you wouldn't get angry; good means you are so happy; good is he is going to help you. That's called "good." You walk out of the office, he helps you carry something; you go there, he opens the door. That's good. Can you do that? You have to really look at it this way and not just say an empty line, that it's good. It's absolutely, a hundred percent understanding what good is.

Headaches – Monthly Migraine Headaches

Every month before my menstrual cycle, I get a migraine headache on the left side of my head. It is extremely painful. Can TCM help me?

Dr. Lu: Yes, there is an excellent chance that TCM can help you, particularly if your headaches are not due to a more serious condition such as a tumor or cancer. The specific treatment will depend on the timing of your headaches—the hour they occur, their frequency and the specific location, among other things.

First, let me say that all headaches are not alike, and they can present a real challenge for TCM practitioners. Six major meridians run through the head. One meridian alone or in combination with the five others can cause a headache. Simple math tells us that TCM recognizes 720 different headaches ($1 \times 2 \times 3 \times 4 \times 5 \times 6 = 720$). This explains why certain medications may work for your headache but not for your husband's or friend's headache. Each of you has a different headache.

The location of headache pain indicates which organs are involved. Headaches that occur at the back of the head are usually related to the Bladder. Pain in the forehead relates to the Stomach. When the Kidney and/or Liver are out of balance, headaches that throb at the top of the head can be experienced.

TCM views migraines like yours that happen every month around menstruation as not just a headache but as a Liver function disorder. In TCM, when we speak about a "function disorder," we mean an energy problem with an organ. Something is not balanced in terms of its energy functions in the body-mind-spirit. The Liver and Gallbladder are partner organs: they share a close energy relationship. This means problems with one organ can strongly affect the other. Headaches on the sides of the head are related to the Gallbladder meridian. This can indicate a problem with this organ's function and by extension, an imbalance in Liver energy. From the TCM viewpoint, all women's health problems are related directly or indirectly to a Liver function disorder, especially if they occur around menstruation. Unless healthy Liver function is restored, these migraines can become chronic. By treating only the symptoms month after month, year after year, this condition actually worsens because the root cause of the problem—unbalanced Liver function—has gone untreated.

With proper diagnosis and natural forms of treatment such as acupuncture and herbal therapy, TCM addresses the source of this issue so the symptom, which is a key sign from your body that something is out of balance, does not return. It is important to know that stress and an excess of emotion, particularly anger, can cause a Liver imbalance. This is because one of that organ's energy functions is to manage the smooth flow of emotion. Learning to manage your emotions and to create a balanced lifestyle that allows for adequate rest and relaxation is essential.

Herbs – Why Chinese Herbal Therapy Is Different

Is there any difference between how Chinese medicine uses herbs and the Western approach?

Dr. Lu: Everything in nature has a special essence, what in TCM is called an "energy essence." This quality has nothing to do with scientific, measurable things like nutritional value or vitamin content. Energy essence describes invisible aspects of a substance: which meridian (or meridians) it travels to, how it affects certain internal organs, and its impact on Qi, or energy, in the body. Energy essence is the property that heals, so Chinese herbal treatments, which are based on this quality, are truly energy treatments. That's one very basic and important principle.

In the West, herbs or herb combinations are often taken based on the symptom the person experiences. Examples of this approach are taking *Dong Quai* for menstrual problems or ginseng for low energy. This way of taking herbs basically substitutes natural substances for chemicals. TCM's approach is very different. The key point is that in the Western method of taking herbs the root cause of the symptom is not addressed. TCM understands that the same symptom in different people can have a very different source. With herbal treatment TCM always seeks to treat the root cause while relieving symptoms, as well as strengthening and protecting any vulnerable organs. These are also fundamental principles of TCM herbal therapy.

With thousands of years of study and practical clinical experience, TCM has vast knowledge of how herbs and many other natural

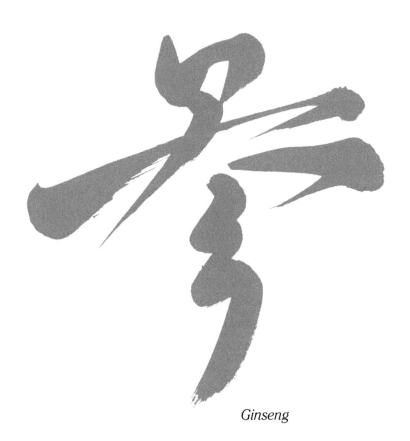

Ginseng

elements work inside the body. This accumulated wisdom extends to how herbs work together in a formula, a unique TCM specialty. In TCM herbal formulas, the individual herbs work together as a team. Each herb has a different function that serves the purpose of the whole formula, and the effect of the sum is greater than that of the parts—the individual herbs used. For example, an herb can be selected for a formula because it is effective at targeting a certain condition or organ. An herb may have a special ability to strengthen the Qi of a certain organ. Or it can help rid the body of unwanted toxic substances or block the movement of the health condition within the body in a certain way. A skilled TCM practitioner knows the herbs, their properties and exactly how they work together. He or she knows that changing just one herb—either adding or removing it—changes the entire formula.

Herbal therapy is one of TCM's great healing resources along with acupuncture, acupressure, Five Element psychology, and Qigong. The whole focus of the TCM approach to herbs is internal, not external, and this creates a very different result than the Western method, in my opinion.

High Blood Pressure

Can high blood pressure be treated with TCM?

Dr. Lu: External symptoms always have a root cause, according to TCM. The true source of any health problem is what TCM practitioners work to determine and treat through their diagnosis and treatment plan. Each person is unique, with his or her own constitution and internal energy (Qi) pattern. It may surprise you to know that from the TCM perspective, similar symptoms do not always have the same root cause.

Take high blood pressure, or hypertension, for example. In the TCM view this condition can be related to the Heart, the Kidney, or the

Stomach organ systems. Frequently it is a combination of organs that have some kind of functional disorder and have fallen into a state of imbalance. Actually, in many cases, you can say that the symptom of high blood pressure is a sign that the entire body is out of balance.

Yin and Yang are two complementary energies that are a part of everything in the universe. They are also part of you. In your body, each has a natural direction: Yin naturally descends and Yang naturally rises. In good health an internal balance is always maintained. Yet with high blood pressure this is not the case. An excess of Qi rises to the head and becomes stuck there. This is why some of the symptoms associated with high blood pressure—headaches, dizziness, redness of the face and eyes—are experienced in the head.

TCM does not treat complex health issues such as high blood pressure in a disease-specific way. This means the TCM treatment approach for this condition has the fundamental understanding that similar symptoms can have very different causes in different people. TCM practitioners carefully analyze individual symptoms and life patterns to determine exactly which organ or organs are out of balance. The practitioner is always looking to find and treat the root cause, so treatment plans for high blood pressure will vary from person to person. This type of healing approach is actually customized for each specific individual.

Western medicine generally approaches this condition by suppressing or controlling symptoms with medication. But in the TCM view, if the root cause of high blood pressure is not addressed—including lifestyle issues—the person can never truly be well. TCM does not separate the symptoms a person experiences from the whole. It seeks to reestablish balance within the body's energy system and then create harmony between the individual and the external natural world.

The symptoms associated with high blood pressure have been successfully treated by TCM for centuries using a variety of natural methods in combination. Acupuncture restores and balances the function of the affected organs. Chinese herbal formulas work to support the organs without negative side effects. Energy practice like Chinese Qigong (energy-building postures and movements) is very beneficial because it helps your organs function more efficiently and at their peak, thereby conserving energy. Because it helps calm the mind and emotions, meditation is also a deeply healing practice. Lifestyle adjustments are also important components in regaining balance and health if you have high blood pressure. Reducing stress and managing the emotions are essential.

Changes in diet—what, when and how you eat—promote healing because food is one of the body's two major sources of energy. Focus on foods with an energy essence that nourishes the unbalanced organs. For the Kidney be sure to include shellfish (clams, lobster, oysters, shrimp and squid), beans (especially black beans), and toasted nuts (pine nuts and walnuts). The Heart benefits from eating broccoli, broccoli rabe and watermelon. Celery, which helps increase Stomach Qi and takes heat out of the body, and zucchini, a vegetable that has a cool essence, both help heal the Stomach. Also, be aware that cold and raw foods unbalance the function of the Stomach. Eat regular meals in a calm, peaceful environment. Just adding these few tips to your daily life on a regular basis can help maximize your healing.

Hormone Replacement Therapy (HRT) – TCM's Unique View

I've been taking hormone replacement therapy for years on the advice of my doctor. Recently there have been more and more stories in the media about the risks of HRT, and now I'm afraid to take it. Is it OK to just stop HRT? What will happen to me once I'm off it, and what's the best course of action for me at this point?

Dr. Lu: When Western doctors prescribe HRT drugs for women who are nearing menopause or who have already started it, their treatment perspective is only looking at one angle of this health issue. The bottom line is this approach doesn't consider a woman's body as a whole—it looks at her body as having a medical condition and treats just the symptoms.

The Western approach hasn't seen that adding chemicals to the body in the form of HRT drugs doesn't balance a woman's hormones; additional ones have just been given from the outside. When the body receives these unnatural hormones, it has to process them. When the body cannot process these hormones, it can cause the internal organs to get even more and more out of balance.

In the Western concept, replacing what is missing (hormones) will restore a woman's body to function so it won't have menopausal symptoms. The TCM understanding is that replacing hormones from the outside will not restore the natural function of a woman's body. Actually, this type of treatment suppresses it. The body's wisdom senses the addition of hormones and gets the message that its own hormone production isn't necessary anymore. TCM believes that if the root causes of menopausal symptoms are not addressed, a woman's body will never function in a healthy way.

One fundamental TCM belief is we are all born with a healing capacity. Women have a unique ability for self-healing because of their menstrual cycle and their special organs: the ovaries and uterus.

It is this inborn capacity that allows women to rebalance and relieve menopausal symptoms without outside hormone therapy. The TCM understanding is that if she has a healthy, balanced body, a woman can produce enough estrogen on her own for her entire life.

From the TCM viewpoint, menopausal symptoms are not caused by the onset of menopause but by the unbalanced state of a woman's body when she begins this natural transition. This is a key point because many of the symptoms Western women experience with their menstrual cycle, often for years, are seen by TCM doctors as signs that a woman's body is out of balance. When these symptoms—PMS, irregular periods, excessive bleeding, breast tenderness, headaches, digestive disturbances, and mood swings, to name just a few—are not addressed, as a woman ages and reaches menopause, they can lead to more serious issues like heart problems or issues involving cysts, tumors, masses and even breast or uterine cancer. TCM's focus on true prevention helps younger women understand that the discomfort they have with their periods is not natural and that effective treatment with natural methods can eventually help them go through menopause and the rest of their life in a healthy, balanced way.

The truth is most women cannot just stop HRT drugs all at once. You have to look at it this way: For many years this kind of problem in a woman's body was never really addressed. The root cause of her health issues at several stages in her life was never treated. That's the whole issue. For women who have been taking HRT, their body hasn't been able to really heal; taking the hormones has made the body function even worse. So you cannot just immediately stop this kind of treatment. You have to slowly get off it.

While gradually stopping HRT, try to find someone using TCM or an alternative medicine approach to help you get your body back into balance. Remember, a healthy body can produce enough hormones for the rest of your life. TCM has had practical clinical experience successfully treating women's health issues for thousands of years. TCM practitioners treat health problems related to menopause with acupuncture and natural herbal therapy, an approach without side effects.

While you slowly go off HRT you still have to do something to help your body gain more energy. Generally, Chinese medicine looks at this health issue as an energy (Qi) deficiency. As we age our energy naturally declines. This is why health problems can start to show when a woman reaches middle age. How can you add to your body's energy supply? It can only come from two sources. One is from the food you eat; the other is from energy practice, like Qigong. These can increase the amount of energy available to balance your body. Without this balance you cannot go on without hormones.

The bottom line is how can a woman achieve balance? There are a couple of issues women have to be concerned with, and these have to be made a priority. Number one is lifestyle. A stressed-out, over-busy lifestyle uses up an enormous amount of energy, so this kind of energy-draining lifestyle has to change. Then the emotions: Women have to consider how to balance their emotions. Anger, worry, stress—these all drain the body's energy supply. Third, the diet has to be changed. These are the outside factors women have to look at.

Women have to consider taking care of their precious health before menopause comes, before disease and illness enter. Why not learn how to keep your body healthy and balanced, so when the time comes you will be able to go through this transition without any struggle? Then you will be able to enjoy the rest of your life in good health. TCM's main concept is prevention. True prevention is the real cure.

Illness that Does Not Heal

I have a problem with my neck. I've been to doctors and specialists; I've had x-rays and MRIs. Apparently there is nothing wrong physically, which doesn't really make sense to me. I try to relax and practice yoga, and I've even had acupuncture. Yet nothing seems to work for me over the long term—I still suffer neck pain. I'm a man in my mid-forties and am in fairly good health otherwise. What do you think is going on?

Dr. Lu: When dealing with this kind of problem—an illness that does not seem to heal despite your best efforts and those of your doctor—you have to look at it in a deep way. It's a difficult concept, very difficult to accept. But the patient has to accept it, and the doctor also has to accept it. No one can treat every illness one hundred percent because sometimes the condition is not a "condition." Sometimes it is karma. This can be particularly difficult for the doctor to accept when he or she really knows what's going on with the patient but still cannot treat the problem effectively.

The first thing we have to accept is that in this world there are many things we cannot see. I believe every condition, whether physical or emotional, is always related to an energy problem. This energy is controlled by a variety of energy systems. Some we can see; some we cannot see. What can be seen depends on the doctor's ability, on his or her level of understanding and how deep he or she can see. Some healers or masters are able to see past lives.

I believe that many things are related to karma. Some health problems appear to be untreatable. This does not mean that they cannot be fixed, but just that the timing is not right. You might need to meet the right person, at the right time, in the right place. Or maybe during this time, instead of focusing on the condition itself, you may need to focus on how to change your body in a deep way, how to

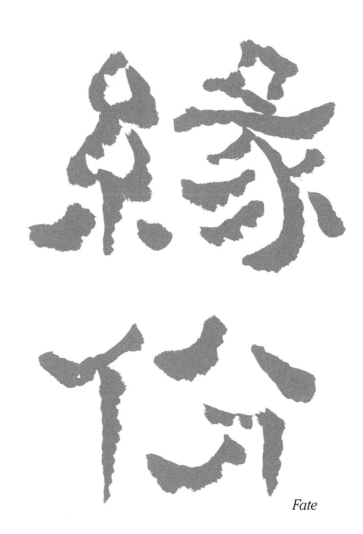

Fate

change not just small things but your whole life.

If karma is operating, it means there is something that you have to recognize. You may have this kind of condition for the rest of your life. But as a result of this condition you will meet different people, you will change your life, your path will change in a spiritual way. And one day, through spiritual development, you may change the karma. If the condition is related to karma, the only way to fix it is through the spiritual path, because no doctor can change karma. No matter how famous the doctor or the master, *you* still have to do the job. They can only help you. Only you can change your own karma by developing your spiritual path.

In your case, because you have been doing positive things to help your health, perhaps you have made your state better, even though you still suffer pain. It's possible that without the efforts you have made, your condition could be worse. So you should be proud of yourself for searching for something. You just have to search a little bit deeper. And don't concentrate only on outside things for help. I believe all the answers were "downloaded" with you before you were born. For every problem or challenge we have, it's important to understand that we also have the answer. All the answers are inside you. The more peaceful you are, the more information you will find out, and the more answers you will get.

Infertility

Can TCM help infertility? My husband and I have been trying to conceive a baby for two years with no luck.

Dr. Lu: TCM has been treating problems of infertility for thousands of years. It understands this condition has two aspects: one has to do with health; the other has to do with fate, which we'll touch on later.

Treating infertility is complicated. This is because it involves trying to create the healthiest body possible in a woman so that a new life will take root and grow. Without a balanced body with organs that work in harmony, it's easy to miscarry. So the first thing a TCM practitioner does is determine how or where a woman's body is out of balance. These physical problems must be addressed first.

Generally speaking, infertility is related to the function of two major organs: the Liver and Kidney. This condition also involves the whole body's health, and other organs can sometimes be involved, including the Stomach, Lung, Heart, and so on. One of the first priorities is to help a woman rebalance her Liver and Kidney functions and then help these organs work in harmony. This provides a better chance of a smooth pregnancy and a healthy baby.

In TCM, the Liver is the most important organ for women's health. So its role in infertility is very important. Controlling the flow of Qi, blood and emotions are three key energy functions of the Liver. This organ is particularly sensitive to stress as well as the emotions of anger and frustration. A busy lifestyle, excessive stress, and chronically held emotions can actually unbalance the function of the Liver. A healthy Liver function is essential to create the best environment for conception. While struggling with infertility, some women become so nervous or so anxious about getting pregnant their bodies refuse to cooperate. There are many stories of couples giving up on having a baby and adopting one, only to find that they become pregnant in a short time.

One of the first clues to infertility that a TCM doctor looks at is the menstrual cycle. If a woman has menstrual difficulties and suffers from symptoms like monthly headaches, nausea, indigestion, PMS and emotional episodes, then any of these symptoms and their root cause must be treated at the beginning.

The goal is to rebalance a woman's cycle so that it comes on time every month, eliminate symptoms and resolve any emotional issues. If she has more serious problems like diabetes or high blood pressure, these problems must also be addressed before considering pregnancy. If not, it's very difficult to deliver the healthiest baby possible. These physical problems can become genetic problems that hide within the newborn. Like a "bad seed," they can appear later if the child's life becomes unbalanced. On the other hand, if the health issues the mother experiences can be fixed, then it is possible for her body to pass along a healing gift to her unborn child.

Of course, infertility does not only relate to the woman. A man's role is also very important. Is he in good health? Are his organs functioning well and in harmony? Is his lifestyle balanced? If not, he also needs to be treated to create optimal health in anticipation of conception.

TCM treats infertility with acupuncture and classical Chinese herbs. Also, TCM can be used as a complement to Western infertility therapies. In my practice, I strongly recommend that the woman and the man meditate or practice Qigong as much as they can. These practices can be very beneficial for conceiving a healthy baby.

Besides the physical reality of pregnancy, there is also an aspect of fate. Sometimes a couple is not meant to get pregnant; it is not their destiny. No matter what they do, nothing works for them. It's possible that their fate may lie in nurturing and raising someone else's child. In the end, receiving another life to guard and grow is in God's hands.

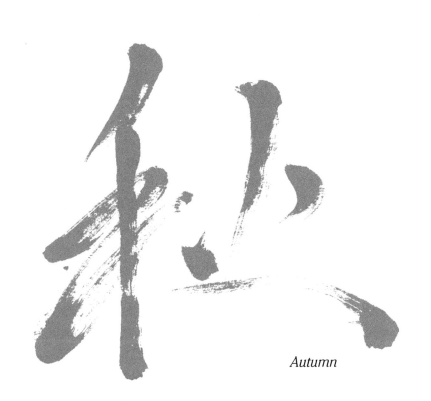

Autumn

Jet Lag

From the TCM perspective, what is going on in the body when you have jet lag?

Dr. Lu: Look at nature: Everything is a circle; everything is a cycle. The seasons change from summer to fall to winter and spring in a cycle every year. This kind of change is easy to see, easy to feel—it is part of the visible. You see the rain come in springtime, flowers grow in summer, leaves fall in autumn, it snows in winter. You can feel the heat, feel the dampness, the dry or cold. Each season has its own special energy, or Qi.

Most people understand Qi as meaning "energy" or "force," as in "life force." This is true but not the whole truth. Qi is more than energy because it also has the qualities of intelligence, message and function. These qualities allow everything in nature to communicate with each other—through Qi. A good example of this is how the Qi of each season communicates with our own body's Qi. You may not realize it or feel it, but still it is happening in your body at a very deep level. Sometimes you do feel it: you may not feel good when the season changes. This means your own Qi is not in harmony with the particular Qi of the new season and therefore cannot make the transition smoothly. Many times an organ is out of balance and causes this kind of seasonal difficulty.

The ancient and timeless Five Element Theory of TCM is one kind of Universal framework that relates and connects everything in the universe in a pattern of five fundamental energies: Wood, Fire, Earth, Metal and Water. In this framework, each season relates to a particular element; each season also has a relationship with a certain organ pair. For example, fall relates to Metal and the Lung, and its partner organ, the Large Intestine.

That's a cycle on the level of the seasons, but did you notice your own body has an internal cycle? Most people don't see this or don't feel this because it's part of the invisible. Even if you don't see or feel it, your body still functions with this cycle every day. Like the seasons, each time of day corresponds with a certain organ. Every two hours, moving around the clock—which is a circle—each of your twelve major internal organs comes into a period where its function, its Qi, is at its strongest. The organ is "in charge" of your body's function at this time. If you experience difficulty every day at the same time of day, chances are there is an imbalance in the specific organ related to that time period. For example, let's say you wake up every night at 3:30 a.m. with some kind of discomfort, maybe even a cough. An experienced TCM doctor would understand this might be a clue pointing to a Lung Qi problem. Why? The Lung comes into its peak function between the hours of 3:00 a.m. and 5:00 a.m.

When we look at jet lag with this deeper understanding of the body's daily internal clock, it's pretty easy to see what is happening. Maybe you live in New Jersey and you are flying to Europe on vacation. The flight leaves at 8:00 p.m. At that time in New Jersey, the Pericardium is the organ in charge. Let's say the flight takes seven hours. That means you arrive in Europe at 3:00 a.m.—just when the Lung is taking over. But what's really happening? It's not 3:00 a.m. in the country where you arrive—where you are—it's six hours ahead on the clock. It's breakfast time! It is 9:00 a.m. and time for the Spleen to go to work helping to digest food.

So the question your body is asking when you have jet lag is which organ is really in charge? In the example above, is it the Lung or the Spleen? This temporary internal confusion creates the symptoms of jet lag: tiredness, a heavy feeling or grogginess, headaches, irritability, irregular sleep pattern or insomnia, constipation or diarrhea.

TCM practitioners use classical Chinese herbal formulas and sometimes acupuncture to help the body process the internal effects of this time change and bring it back into balance.

The Daily Internal Clock

Lung	3:00 a.m. – 5:00 a.m.
Large Intestine	5:00 a.m. – 7:00 a.m.
Stomach	7:00 a.m. – 9:00 a.m.
Spleen	9:00 a.m. – 11:00 a.m.
Heart	11:00 a.m. – 1:00 p.m.
Small Intestine	1:00 p.m. – 3:00 p.m.
Bladder	3:00 p.m. – 5:00 p.m.
Kidney	5:00 p.m. – 7:00 p.m.
Pericardium	7:00 p.m. – 9:00 p.m.
Triple Warmer*	9:00 p.m. – 11:00 p.m.
Gallbladder	11:00 p.m. – 1:00 a.m.
Liver	1:00 a.m. – 3:00 a.m.

* In TCM the Triple Warmer coordinates the flow between the upper, middle and lower areas of the body.

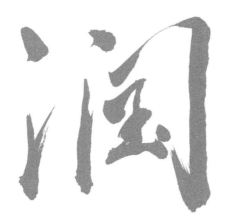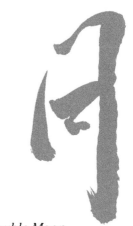

Double Moon

Joy – Choose Joy to Get What You Want

What is the best way to deal with the suffering that comes from illness?

Dr. Lu: Suffering is one kind of power because it draws all the attention: give me love, give me care. Look at it like a business: Is there profit or loss? Is the suffering and the pain worth it? If you are suffering, you get some benefit there. What is it? Through suffering you may get what you want, but this is not the only way. It's a choice you make. Why not choose joy to get what you want? You can have a happy life, enjoy your life and still get what you want. One second, one phone call, can break the suffering, just like one night of the full moon can balance the other thirty days of the month. So try to do more things that make you happy.

Menopause – An Energy Gateway for Women

Since I started menopause I've had very intense symptoms: hot flashes, mood swings and insomnia are the worst of them. Can TCM provide any relief or is this just what a woman has to go through at this time of life?

Dr. Lu: It's interesting; the word "menopause" isn't even in the TCM vocabulary. If you look in every classical traditional Chinese medical text, you won't find it. What you will find are references to the symptoms women experience when they reach this life transition. Actually, TCM calls these symptoms "menstrual cycle ending symptoms." So you may be surprised to learn that menopause is essentially a Western concept.

The TCM concept is that women have a menstrual cycle and it has a beginning and an end. It's a natural part of a woman's life; it's nature's way. From the beginning to the end of this life cycle, if a woman is healthy her menstruation will be regular and free of any problems.

But if a woman is in poor health and her internal energy, or Qi, is not balanced, her body will express this internal condition through many menstrual symptoms: irregular periods, PMS, painful periods, breast tenderness, headaches, fever during cramps, to name just a few.

When I began practicing TCM in the West many years ago, I was surprised to find out that most Western women accept these menstrual symptoms as "normal." The TCM view is that over time, chronic symptoms like these can lead to more serious problems like the formation of masses, tumors and even cancer, if left untreated. And women who have these menstrual symptoms regularly most likely will have problems like the ones you describe when they reach the age when their cycle begins to end or stops altogether. You might think back and remember if you had any of these difficulties during the years you had your cycle. The disturbing symptoms some women experience during menopause are not really the result of menopause but the condition of their bodies before they reach this transition.

One fundamental TCM principle is prevention. This means the good news is women can learn to take care of themselves and achieve good health with an understanding of how to increase and balance their internal energy. Time-tested, effective TCM healing techniques like acupuncture, herbal therapy, Qigong (a Chinese self-healing energy practice) and lifestyle changes offer women the support to accomplish this. Women who have already reached menopause can also benefit from natural care without medication and its problematic side effects. It's never too late to improve your health.

When you work with a TCM practitioner, he or she will treat the symptoms you have, providing relief, while addressing the root cause of your condition. It's important to know that as we age our Qi naturally declines. This means we have less energy to "spend" doing our normal daily routine. If no adjustment is made for this energy gap, your body and its organs will be affected. Kidney energy deficiency is, in TCM's understanding, one root cause of menopausal issues. Kidney energy powers the many functions of the body. When it is weak or deficient, eventually all the organs and a woman's overall health will suffer.

Another organ that is important is the Liver—the number one organ in terms of women's health. Why is it number one? The Liver controls the smooth flow of everything—blood, Qi and emotions—in the body. Women need to understand the role chronic stress and anger (the emotion that resonates with the Liver) play in creating illness. Balance between work and rest, and in what a woman eats—and when—are also key factors.

TCM believes everyone is born with a self-healing ability. Women particularly have a unique ability to heal because of their menstrual cycle and their special organs: the uterus and the ovaries. These give them the capacity to create wellness so their body can function in a healthy way—at any age. TCM sees menopause as a deep energy shift that goes beyond physical changes. It's a natural and normal part of a woman's life, yet it has the power to affect her mind, emotions and spirit. Menopause is a gateway, a unique opportunity for a woman to prepare her body, mind and spirit for a healthy, long life. It's a time for new beginnings as she becomes free to pursue or complete her life's mission.

Men's Health – Prostate Issues

I'm in my early sixties and I'm starting to have prostate problems. Can TCM help me?

Dr. Lu: Would it surprise you to know that classical traditional Chinese medical texts outlined successful treatments for prostate problems as long as one thousand years ago? From the TCM perspective, one of the major causes of prostate problems is Kidney energy deficiency.

Many times this energy, or Qi, deficiency is caused by too much sex, particularly from the time when the man was young.

In TCM theory the Kidney controls all functions related to sexual activity and reproduction. Kidney energy is the fuel that powers the functions of your whole body. As we age our Kidney energy naturally declines. When it's gone, that's it—it's our time to die. Sex draws on the energy of the Kidney. When Kidney energy is overused—which is the case when there's too much sexual activity at any age—the prostate gland cannot receive enough energy circulation to keep it healthy and functioning smoothly. To most people in the West, where frequent sexual activity from a young age is fairly common, this is a concept that seems almost unbelievable. Yet it is a basic TCM understanding that less sex means increased Kidney Qi, which is the energy foundation for a long and healthy life. So part of the treatment for prostate issues includes moderation in sexual activity or even abstinence, particularly if the man is very young or if his general state of health is weak.

It's not unusual for a prostate condition to be accompanied by other physical problems. High cholesterol, high blood pressure, heart disease, depression and nervousness are just a few of the many health issues that can be present with a prostate condition. These problems often cause prostate problems to show up more quickly. TCM targets these other conditions for treatment first to see if it improves the prostate. In TCM theory, the conditions are reciprocal: treating one can improve the other.

An effective way to treat prostate problems is with Chinese herbs. Modern TCM practitioners use classical herbal formulas that have been used for this health problem with success for thousands of years. Acupuncture is also used to rebalance the body's energy. Surgery, according to TCM, is not a good solution because its effects are short-term, and it does nothing to address the problem's real source: Kidney energy deficiency.

Men's Health – Sexual Function

Do you believe it is healthy for men to take medications that enhance sexual performance?

Dr. Lu: Modern men have a number of different health issues, including sexual function problems. The lifestyle causes of these health problems may be new, but the ways to treat their source—imbalances in energy—have been successfully used by Chinese medicine practitioners for thousands of years.

In Chinese medicine we believe male energy moves in eight-year cycles. Every eight years men complete one more cycle. Around age 8 permanent teeth grow in. From age 8 to age 16, a big change happens: boys mature into men who can reproduce. In terms of energy, generally speaking, after this age it's a downward slope. This means at age 16, men have reached the highest energy level they will have in their life. Why? It relates to Kidney energy, which naturally declines as we age. So when we look at men's health issues, particularly when it comes to aging, we always look at Kidney function. Without this organ in good shape energy-wise, it's impossible for men to be strong and have good health.

The Kidney's main function, in TCM, is to store energy and supply power for your whole body. It's one of your body's two major sources of life force, or energy. (The other is energy received from the process of digesting food.) This kind of energy you inherit from your parents— all your genetic power is stored in the Kidney. After you are born, this energy is used for growth throughout your body. All growth—including sexual development, the production of hormones, and the ability to reproduce—is totally related to your Kidney Qi.

Men should understand that overdoing the amount of sex they have can lead to a Kidney problem and prostate issues. The other thing is thinking about sex all the time. Yes, *thinking* about it! Remember that everything is about energy. The mind is so powerful; it has energy. So thinking about sex is essentially the same as having sex. Every time you daydream about sex you make the energy circulate in the whole prostate area. The trouble is the energy gets stuck there because it doesn't get released by having sex. A lot of men think about sex many times during the day. If you're constantly thinking about it, the energy goes there all the time and the prostate never gets a rest. It's like an elastic band that gets pulled and pulled: it stretches and stretches and gets bigger. Sooner or later it won't have power anymore.

So to answer your specific question: What about taking Western medications that give an erection or prolong the amount of time men can have sex? Chinese medicine believes this is not good for the health of men's bodies as a whole. Stimulating an erection in this way will only allow you to use energy you don't really have. It's like borrowing money from a credit card and going to Atlantic City to try and make money! It will eventually cause a Kidney deficiency and damage both your Kidney and Liver. In TCM all the organs are interrelated. The Kidney supports the Liver; it generates energy for the Liver and has a mother/child relationship with it. This means when your Kidney energy is low it will eventually affect your Liver function. Once the mother is exhausted, the child will suffer. If a man cannot get an erection naturally, it means that his Kidney energy is low and needs healing support.

Chinese medicine treats men's health issues with natural methods that create good health and leave no damaging side effects for the body to deal with. Prevention is the true specialty of traditional Chinese medicine, so we educate men about the benefits of natural healing techniques and balanced lifestyle choices so they can build and then maintain their health. Qigong is a very powerful healing practice because it actually builds Kidney Qi. Men should understand that they are responsible for their own health.

Menstruation – Sex during Menstruation

My boyfriend wants to have sex with me even when I have my period, but I don't feel comfortable having sex then. What does TCM say about this?

Dr. Lu: From an energy point of view, TCM does not advise having intercourse while a woman has her period. This is because during this time a woman is particularly vulnerable and it is easier for her to develop a health problem. And from an energy standpoint, any problem can be more easily transferred to her partner. Sexual diseases also can be readily transferred from one partner to the other when a woman is menstruating.

Women who have symptoms such as yeast infections, blood infections, urinary tract infections, discharge and fibroids should be careful because their body is already showing signs of an energy deficiency and energy imbalance. PMS, menstrual cramping, breast tenderness and headaches are all signs of a Liver function disorder; women who have these symptoms should be especially careful during their period because at that time it is easier to create an emotional imbalance or cause a Liver energy deficiency imbalance.

If a problem were created during this time most likely it would be very difficult to fix because the problem would go beyond the physical level to a functional imbalance, an energy imbalance. Having sex during the period might cause a menstrual cycle disorder which could show up in symptoms such as painful periods, cramping and longer periods, or in other signs such as chronic lower abdomen pain and nausea—many chronic conditions that a woman would not necessarily relate to having sex during menstruation. If a woman does have one of these conditions and has not been successful in finding a diagnosis through Western tests, or effective treatment, she might think back and discover that the symptom relates to sex during the period. If this

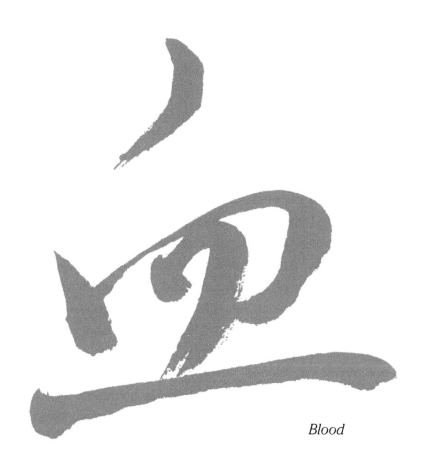

Blood

is the situation, acupuncture and Chinese herbs would be the only way to readjust the woman's energy.

It's important for women to be peaceful, to rest and recover during their period. In TCM theory, blood is the "mother" of Qi (vital energy) and Qi is the commander of blood. This means that blood and Qi have a very close relationship. Blood provides nutrients for the movement of Qi; Qi is in blood, so that when blood is lost, energy is lost too. On the other hand, Qi is essential for making blood. When a woman is menstruating, her body is going through a unique process: she loses blood and with the blood, energy. So her focus at this time of the month should be on recovering energy, not expending it. Quiet activities such as meditation are best at this time.

Menstruation – Swimming during Menstruation

I have a friend who is Chinese, and she says that in China women do not swim when they have their period. Is this a cultural custom or are there real medical reasons to avoid swimming when menstruating?

Dr. Lu: First, I will say a few important things about menstruation from the energy perspective. Based on TCM's understanding, a woman's body goes through an energy change during her menstrual cycle: blood is stored and then the body creates an energy flow to discharge this blood. A woman needs a healthy body to make enough blood every month for a proper menstrual flow. According to TCM, three major organs relate to menstruation: the Liver, the Kidney and the Spleen. Problems with periods can be a sign that any one or a combination of these organs is having an energy function problem.

It takes extra energy to menstruate, so women should try to save as much energy as possible during their periods. This means resting and taking it easy at this time. Also, it's better for women to avoid strenuous exercise while they have their period—intense workouts will make it harder to recover. Fatigue is often a symptom when a woman exercises too much while menstruating. A balanced and healthy approach involves more gentle movement such as Taiji, simple stretching or walking.

The reason TCM advises women not to swim during menstruation is that their body is more sensitive and very vulnerable at this time. So it's smart for a woman to be careful and protect herself. Any situation that could bring water into the vagina should be avoided because in most cases the water is not perfectly clean. Swimming pools can carry bacteria and are generally full of chemicals; even the ocean is not pure anymore. And even if a woman wears a tampon she is not protected—the cotton of the tampon can absorb water.

It's important to understand that disease brought into the body during a woman's period can go deep and create problems that later on will be difficult to treat. For example, while swimming during her period, a woman could be more vulnerable to getting an infection which could later cause chronic problems such as yeast infections, menstrual cramps, vaginal discharge and urinary tract infection. When women swim during their menstrual cycle, frequently they can experience leg cramping, a condition they might not connect to swimming during their period.

Swimming and bathing (it's better to take a shower, not a bath) should be avoided from the day before the start of the period through the last day. Also, do not douche during this time. Women who feel the need to take a hot bath to reduce discomfort during menstruation can instead apply a hot water bottle or a heating pad to the abdomen.

Osteoporosis

How does TCM treat osteoporosis? I'm a middle-aged woman who has been diagnosed with this condition.

Dr. Lu: TCM is all about relationships—relationships and energy. Today we know from quantum physics that everything is energy. For thousands of years TCM has understood the relationships between humans and nature; between the body, mind and spirit; between the organs and different areas of the body. TCM's Five Element Theory is one kind of master "blueprint" that organizes all natural phenomena into five essential patterns: Wood, Fire, Earth, Metal and Water. Each element is related to a season, a climate type, a pair of internal organs, an area of the body, an emotion, an aspect of the soul, sound, taste, color . . . the associations are limitless. And everything is connected by Qi, by energy.

When someone has a health problem and shows a symptom, we treat the symptom, but we also look deeper for the source of the symptom, what TCM calls the "root cause." Without addressing the root cause, the treatment will not produce lasting results. The problem may even go somewhere else in the body or show up later in a different form. If this happens, later on, a good TCM doctor can always trace it back to the original problem.

Osteoporosis is a condition that relates to the bones. In TCM we know the bones are related to the Kidney. Everybody is born with a source of energy they inherit from their parents. This is called "Inborn Qi," and it is stored in the Kidney. Inborn Qi is like an energy "savings account." How much energy you get and what quality it has you can't change. What you can control is how you manage that savings account.

As we age our Qi naturally declines. When it's gone we have reached the end of our time here on Earth. Women have seven-year energy cycles. Between their sixth and seventh cycles (between the

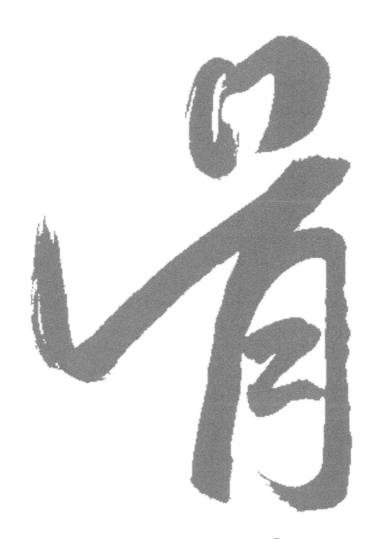

Bone

ages of 42 and 49) most women begin menopause. If she has taken pretty good care of herself up to this point, a woman can make this transition smoothly. If she has had a busy, overstressed life, problems may start to show; maybe they have even started to show before this time but have gone untreated. When women reach the age of menopause their Qi level drops and this is when signs of aging can appear. As you age, how you take care of yourself can make the decline in energy less dramatic.

There are several areas of the body that the Kidney "controls." This means Kidney energy supports the overall health of these areas. The ears, the hair on your head, the bones (including the teeth, which TCM calls the "surplus of the bone"), the knees and the lower back (where the physical kidneys are located) all relate to the Kidney organ system. It also is in charge of sexual function and reproduction. So when symptoms appear in these places on the body or with these functions, it shows some kind of Kidney problem. Most of the time it relates to a Kidney Qi deficiency—this is the case with osteoporosis. The Kidney doesn't have the energy to nourish the bones, and they become weak and brittle. The following health problems indicate a Kidney Qi deficiency: earaches, ringing in the ears (tinnitus), hearing loss, a feeling all the time of cold on the inside, hair loss, teeth problems, knee pain and lower back pain, and loss of sex drive.

For treatment of osteoporosis and these other issues, TCM doctors generally build Kidney energy with acupuncture and herbal therapy. Qigong, an ancient Chinese energy practice, is an excellent way to build your health because it helps the organs work more efficiently, and this helps your body save energy in the long run. Eating balanced and healthy meals also can improve your health. Food is a very good resource and it's relatively cheap. There are many foods that nourish the Kidney: walnuts, pine nuts, black beans, seafood—especially shellfish, and especially for osteoporosis, try making an old-fashioned bone soup. Elements nourish like elements: animal bones used in a soup can help strengthen your bones.

Outside Reflects the Inside

My boyfriend says I tend to be too "negative." He says I complain too much about some of the people I meet and have to work with. I guess I do complain a lot—other people have said the same thing to me. Is there something you can say to someone (me) who is frustrated most of the time with the way some people are?

Dr. Lu: The most important thing here is to know that we create our own reality. What does that really mean? On a deep level we set up the "box of signs" of what we want to see. We may want evidence that someone loves us: they call after work, bring the milk home, and things like that. If we are looking for love, we search to see all the evidence that the person loves us. If we want to see the opposite, we search for the proof that confirms that view. But it's our mind that sets up the box of limits that proves what we really want to see.

Buddhists use a different language to say the same thing. For example, they say that everything on the outside is a reflection of what's inside. We only see what we know; we only see what's in our consciousness. As we get to know someone, we see what is similar to us, and if there is enough similarity, we put them in the "I like" category. We have to have an open mind to explore someone who is dissimilar. They are there for a reason; perhaps they are a gate for something beyond what we know. There's got to be something behind the dissimilarity. The person who hates someone—behind the hate is something powerful. We need to open our mind and believe in change, and then something we don't know will help us move into the unknown.

Parasites

I'm an American businessman who travels frequently. I'm worried about getting parasites while in some of the countries I visit. I have read that TCM can treat this problem with only natural methods. Is this true?

Dr. Lu: Generally speaking, Americans are particularly vulnerable to parasites because many suffer from Stomach function problems. This means that from an energy perspective their Stomach function is un-balanced and too weak to fight off these kinds of toxic invaders. Also, stress, a factor experienced by many people in this society, further compromises a person's ability to avoid this type of health issue or heal once they have it.

You might have read that TCM has been treating disease caused by parasites for nearly two thousand years. As early as the third cen-tury C.E., the Chinese doctor Zhang Zhongjing discussed pinworms in his work *Treatise on Febrile Diseases*. And in his writings in the early seventh century C.E., Chao Yuanfang detailed pinworm and tapeworm infestations and cited their causes: unhygienic diet, and in the case of tapeworms, eating undercooked meat. Ancient Chinese doctors were also well aware of the dangers of drinking contaminated water. They knew how to effectively treat the health issues that arise with parasites.

TCM uses herbal therapy to treat this problem. It works first to expel the parasite from the body and then to strengthen the body so internal conditions are not hospitable to the parasite and it cannot return. For example, when dealing with a blood parasite, TCM would target treatment for the Heart, Liver and brain since all three share integral relationships with the blood. Herbal formulas would be used to stimulate the blood's energy, which would produce antibodies to kill the parasites and prevent them from reproducing. Once the body's immune system is strengthened, herbs like ginger, garlic and pumpkin seed can help maintain a healthy internal environment.

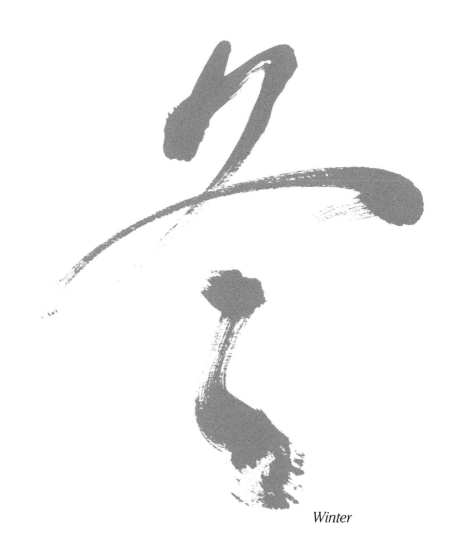

Winter

Prevention really is the best cure, so it would be smart for you to build up and balance your Stomach energy and immune system while you have the chance, particularly if they are showing any signs of weakness. Digestive disturbances like abdominal pain and distension, gas, belching and diarrhea are signs from the body that can indicate that the Stomach function is out of balance. Food is one of the main sources of energy for your body, so a quality diet is very important. Try to eat healthy foods and regular meals. Avoid foods that unbalance the Qi (energy) of your Stomach, such as raw foods and cold foods and beverages. Energy practices like Qigong can help build your Qi and immune system and help you manage stress, so they also can benefit your body as a whole.

Pine Pollen

I have a close friend who is a patient of yours. She says you have suggested she take pine pollen as a supplement. What is it used for?

Dr. Lu: Pine pollen is one of nature's special healing materials. The purpose of taking herbs and natural supplements like pine pollen is to connect to the message of nature through the particular substance.

Pine trees are so unique. Why don't they drop their needles in winter? Why do they stay green through the coldest weather? In winter, if you want to stay alive you need more energy. Pine trees have the most energy because they can fight the cold and even stay green. Other plants have to drop their leaves. When you take pine pollen, you get its message. You become part of this evergreen strength: no fear, green in winter, forever you.

Pine pollen is extra special because you cannot harvest the pollen every year. You have to wait about twenty years to harvest it. So

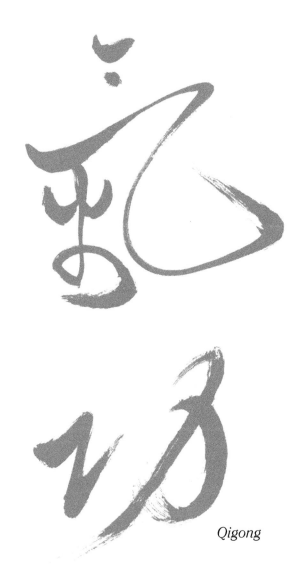

Qigong

pine pollen represents not only the highest energy of the season but the highest energy of nature. If the pine tree didn't meet the energy requirement of nature, then it wouldn't have pollen.

For thousands of years TCM has understood and used the healing properties of the pine tree. In terms of healing the body, pine pollen is very good for the skin and it benefits cardio health. The pine tree is also used to treat arthritis. Pine sap traditionally has been used in cancer treatment in China. Pine nuts are a very healthy food. Their essence travels to the Lung and Kidney meridians, and TCM practitioners advise patients to use pine nuts in their diet to strengthen the Kidney and to help relieve constipation. Pine pollen and other pine tree materials are not used so much in the West, but in China they are considered one of the most powerful natural substances.

Qigong – Building Health with Qigong

How does practicing Qigong help maintain good health?

Dr. Lu: Qigong is an ancient and very powerful Chinese self-healing practice. It is truly the basis of TCM. Many people are not aware of what Qigong can really do. Otherwise everybody would practice it— every day! Qigong has the ability to connect body, mind and spirit so they work together in harmony. TCM understands that when these dimensions of being function well together, you have a fundamental condition for good health. Qigong builds and balances your internal energy, your Qi. It also helps to strengthen your body's own healing ability. Everyone is born with this skill, but sometimes because of a person's lifestyle or because of illness this self-healing capability grows dormant. Qigong is the strongest medicine, but it must be used wisely because it affects your energy body.

Think of your body's energy reserve as a bank account. Just living can deplete this account, your Qi. You need to keep building it up so that you are not left with too little energy for your body to function well. The more you practice Qigong, the greater your Qi reserves will be. That's if you don't waste the energy you have accumulated. Modern life is difficult. Whatever energy reserves you can gain with even twenty minutes of daily Qigong practice, you have a lot of places you have to spend that energy—body, mind and spirit—in your daily life. It's a high interest rate!

TCM theory says that if you have sufficient Qi and your organs work in harmony, you will have good health. The more you practice Qigong, each of your organs will work more efficiently. They will also work better as a team, which saves your body a great deal of energy. To use a car as an analogy: A car that is well-tuned will work better and use less fuel than one in poor condition.

When you practice Qigong in a dedicated way, your practice will deepen and you will experience many things, many miracles. You will discover your own healing power. Your intuition will open up and grow. Then you are mentally and emotionally free.

Qigong – Faith Is the Foundation of Qigong

What is the foundation of Qigong?

Dr. Lu: The foundation of Qigong is absolute faith. Everything rests on uncovering this faith in your heart. There can be no personal transformation, no real change, without this faith. It is a faith that believes anything is possible; that anything can happen at any time; that horizons are boundless; that human life is meant for a destiny far beyond what our minds can imagine. When you have this kind of faith, there is nothing you cannot accomplish. And it is this faith that gives you the hope to keep trying, even when things seem hopeless.

Rosacea

I am a woman in my late forties and in the last couple of years I have developed rosacea—the skin on my nose and cheeks is red and blotchy all the time. How does TCM treat this problem?

Dr. Lu: TCM sees rosacea as a condition caused by a Liver and Stomach function disorder. These two organs are not functioning in harmony at the level of energy. Generally it is a Liver function disorder that causes Stomach function problems. The Liver is responsible for "controlling" the Stomach, which means that if the Stomach's energy is in excess the Liver is able to adjust or moderate it. But sometimes, if the Liver's energy is too strong it can "attack" the Stomach: the excess Liver energy flows to the Stomach, causing a Stomach energy dysfunction. Everything is interrelated. When the nose shows a red color it means the Stomach has an excess; the Stomach's energy has stagnated and a lot of heat is generated. This heat is then reflected on the face and nose.

There are signals that the body gives when it's on a path toward this condition. People who suffer from this problem might first experience bad breath, heartburn, constipation, and in women, a problem with their menstrual cycle. These are all signs of a Liver function disorder; they show there is already energy stagnation. The idea is that people suffer from stress, anger, or some kind of emotional disorder, and these states prevent the Liver energy from flowing.

From the Western perspective rosacea is difficult to treat. According to TCM understanding, this difficulty is experienced because

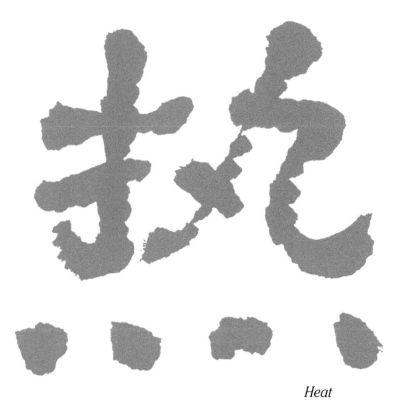

Heat

the root cause of the problem is not treated. Western doctors don't treat the Liver; they concentrate only on the skin. Unfortunately, treating just the skin will never fix this kind of problem. The red and blotchy skin is only a sign, the outcome of the root cause of the problem. TCM doesn't focus on the skin; it focuses on helping to smooth and harmonize Liver and Stomach function because the energy is stuck there.

TCM uses acupuncture and herbal therapy to treat rosacea. Other important factors are lifestyle and diet: these have to change to see lasting improvement. Because stress is often a key element in this type of condition, effort must be made to reduce stress and maintain emotional balance. People who have rosacea can also greatly benefit by modifying their diet in several ways. They should stay away from foods that create more heat in the body: meat, dairy products such as cheese, spicy foods, and fried or barbecued foods. There are many foods that are very helpful in cooling the body down, and TCM practitioners "prescribe" them to individuals with rosacea. For example, bean sprouts and celery are two foods with a cooling essence.

Sports Injuries

I am an avid skier, and every winter by the end of the season, my knees are sore and somewhat painful. A couple of years ago I twisted my right knee very badly while skiing. I immediately applied ice to it, yet this knee grows worse with time: it aches and seems to be weaker. My doctor has been advising surgery. What can TCM do for this type of problem?

Dr. Lu: Generally speaking, sports injuries fall into two categories. In one, the tendon is injured—the tendon and muscle are overstretched and hurt. This kind of injury will cause motion problems; the body has limited motion and the person will experience pain. The other category involves injury to the bone, such as a broken bone. In the first case, if the injury does not involve any damage to the bone, acupuncture and *tui na* (Chinese acupressure) can help. In my experience, with knee injuries, sometimes just one or two good treatments can bring about an immediate change in many patients, and without surgery.

For example, if you experience difficulty in bending the knee or if walking down stairs hurts, try to massage a point on the inside of the lower thigh, just above the knee. (To find this spot, place your hand with the fingers covering the knees; where the thumb naturally rests is the right spot. It is often sore.) With knee injuries, most people experience a problem in this area, and by massaging it the difficulty is often released. You may feel the tendon to be very tight. By gently massaging it, you can release the pain. Also, you can massage the area with some wine, whiskey, gin, tiger balm, or even Tabasco sauce. These items help to stimulate the circulation. Drinking a small amount of wine can also help the injury.

From the TCM perspective, any kind of injury involves blood stagnation. In order to help the blood flow you need to increase the flow of Qi, or energy, so acupuncture and herbs are used. It is important not to use ice for an injury. In the martial arts, heat is used on sports injuries. In the short term, using ice may be better than heat because you will feel immediate relief from the pain. However, ice will keep everything in the area frozen, making the circulation worse and possibly causing arthritis later on. Good treatment—good acupuncture, good acupressure—is much more effective than ice because it treats the root cause of the problem.

One fundamental principle in TCM states that everything that happens on the outside of the body reflects an imbalance on the inside. In your case, with knee difficulties, the knees represent the Kidney. TCM theory states that the Kidney "governs" the knees. This means the state of a person's Kidney energy is reflected in the condition of their knees, along with other areas of the body. A knee issue is a sign that you have a Kidney function disorder and a Kidney energy deficiency. In other words, with a healthy Kidney you'd never get a knee problem. That part of your body is vulnerable for a reason. A person with a healthy body might fall, but he or she would never get an injury. A person with a truly healthy, balanced body would never fall. If you fall, it means there is some imbalance. There are no accidents!

Many times it looks like the difficulty is in the ligaments, but the problem lies in the muscles and tendons. If you help the muscle and the tendon release the blood stagnation, it can help the entire area to heal. The fundamental concept is that as long as energy can flow, there will be no injury and no pain. Before resorting to more drastic treatments, you should begin with TCM and seek a local acupuncturist/herbalist to help you strengthen your Kidney function. Often, if the treatment is right, it can help you avoid surgery.

Spring Offers a Special Opportunity

What can I do to build my health in spring?

Dr. Lu: Every year, spring is the most important season of the whole year. Take this special opportunity. Try to change your level of health in spring. Look at nature: Everything is growing and flowing in spring. If you plant a seed too late, the plant won't grow; if you plant it too early, it won't grow—it will wither. Nature is not unbalanced. If you haven't cleaned up all your internal "garbage" from the last year by spring, the coming year will be difficult. By garbage I mean internal things: energy that is blocked or stuck and issues that need to be let go.

Eat well; eat more good food. Use the essence of food to help

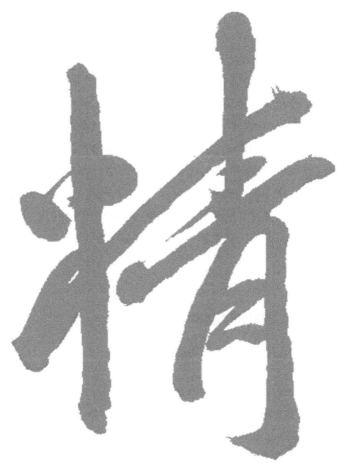

Essence

you. If you eat well, you won't have to take herbs. This way is best because food is more basic. There is a traditional Taoist maxim that illustrates this principle: "Food is better than herbs, Qi (internal energy) is better than food, and emptiness (a state of harmony with the Universal) is better than Qi." Try to eat something that will naturally help you in terms of your diet. There are many foods that benefit the Liver, the organ associated with spring, according to the Five Element Theory. Scallions, bitter greens like dandelions and broccoli rabe, bamboo shoots, fennel, garlic, ginger, and lemon have an energy essence that helps heal the Liver.

If you take care of yourself really well in spring you shouldn't get sick during the other seasons. In my experience, when a person has a health problem, if you trace it back you can find that something happened in the spring—be it physical, emotional or spiritual. The Liver is the organ responsible for the flow of blood, Qi and emotions in your body. Go with the flow to stay in harmony with the season.

Tinnitus (Ringing in the Ears)

In the past month I have started to get ringing in my ears. Is there something TCM can do to help this condition? I am a musician in my mid-fifties.

Dr. Lu: If your physical ear does not have a problem—tests show that there is no actual damage to the ear—tinnitus or ringing sounds in the ears is related to what TCM calls a function disorder. This is an energy problem. According to TCM's Five Element Theory the ear is considered the "gateway" or opening of the Kidney. Another way of putting this concept is that the ear is a sort of Kidney "energy detector." If your Kidney energy (Qi) is deficient, much like a home smoke detector when there's smoke or fire, your ears (either one or both) will have a sound. The louder and the longer the duration of sound, the lower your Kidney energy is. Sometimes, people with this problem experience a decrease in the loudness or the length of time it is present when they sleep well and are more rested.

For musicians, it may appear that the sound is caused by exposure to loud music, but in reality the cause is most likely due to constantly working late nights. TCM understands that when the body is forced to work and be active at night, particularly past midnight when it is natural for the body to rest, it expends many more times—double or triple—the amount of energy than it does during the day. It is like swimming against the current. When you live like this over a long period of time, you are continually "spending" your Kidney Qi. Once it goes below a certain level, your body sends you a signal—it sets off a kind of alarm—and that is the ringing in your ears. This is the body's attempt to tell you it needs a refill, the tank is getting empty.

The real way to fix this kind of health problem is to change your lifestyle. The bottom line is if you don't change, later on things will only get worse. Kidney energy is what powers the body, and without a sufficient amount, all your organs will eventually suffer because they are interrelated and interdependent. If this problem is caught while it is not too serious, you can regenerate and accumulate your energy. It will just take some time. Kidney energy is like money: it's difficult to save and very easy to spend.

TCM doctors have effectively treated tinnitus for centuries using natural healing techniques. Acupuncture is very beneficial to balance and harmonize organ function. There are several classical herbal formulas that are very helpful for this condition, and they must be taken for at least a few months. Qigong (self-healing energy postures and movements) is extremely beneficial because it helps increase and balance your Qi. This maximizes the function of your internal organs, thereby saving energy.

Another treatment that can help is to use small magnets. Tape them to the bottom of the foot over a special energy point located at the center of each foot, near the ball, and in line with the second toe. Wear the magnets daily for at least a couple of months. This can stimulate the Kidney.

And last but not least, lifestyle changes. To totally heal this kind of problem, you need to constantly save your energy, and this is difficult to do, particularly living a busy Western lifestyle. You have to learn the value of regular rest and relaxation. Also, learn to let difficulties go emotionally—constant churning of emotions burns up your energy. It's also important to know that overdoing it in terms of sex is not good. Kidney energy is lost during sex, so approach it with moderation in mind. Treatment with a good TCM practitioner can definitely help you with this problem.

Toenail Fungus

I haven't had much lasting success with Western treatments for my toenail fungus. I've even tried herbal treatments from the health food store without any success. Can TCM treat this condition with long-term results?

Dr. Lu: The treatments you've tried haven't worked because they do not address the root cause of your problem. Western treatments—drug therapy and even the latest laser treatments—focus on the nail itself. The herbal treatments you mentioned also approach the problem from the outside in: they try to kill the fungus "attacking" the nail. But working from the outside in will never achieve long-term results for this health issue because it is caused by an internal energy imbalance. Unless this imbalance is corrected, any external treatments are not going to work for very long. That's why these kinds of treatments are basically temporary: they need to be repeated over and over to make the results last. And most of the time, you never really get healthy looking nails.

The root cause of nail fungus is a Liver energy imbalance. In TCM the nails—both the fingernails and toenails—are related to the Liver. The Liver is responsible for the condition of the tendons, and the nails are considered an outgrowth or "surplus" of the tendons. So you can't really have healthy nails and tendons without a healthy Liver.

One of the Liver's main jobs is storing blood, which nourishes both the tendons and nails. Problems with the nails, including cracked, dry, brittle nails, and toenail fungus, are actually signs from the body that the Liver has an energy function disorder. An experienced TCM practitioner would determine exactly how your Liver is imbalanced and treat it with acupuncture and classical herbal formulas that you take internally. This treatment approach works from the inside out to restore the balance of your body. And the effects are long-lasting once the Liver is balanced and you maintain that state. Also, a balanced lifestyle and healthy diet can help keep your body well.

TMJ (Temporomandibular Joint Disorder)

I have a problem with TMJ. Frequently I wake up in the morning with tremendous tension in my jaw and face and sometimes even a bad headache. I have been reading about the causes of TMJ, and various authors differ on the cause: from injury to allergies to certain bite problems. What does TCM see as the cause of TMJ and how do you treat it?

Dr. Lu: There are many different ideas on what causes a TMJ disorder: for instance, trauma from accidents, stress and some of the other causes you have mentioned. From the TCM perspective, and in my opinion, TMJ is related to a Stomach function disorder as well as a disorder of the Stomach meridians (the meridians of the organs run on both sides of the body). The first thing we see is that the Stomach meridians run through the jaw area. Because of stress and an energy imbalance, the Stomach's energy stagnates—something is stuck—and then this area of the body will show the effects of that stagnation.

The reason that clenching, grinding and TMJ show up at night is because during the day the conscious mind is busy, distracted; its attention is turned to different things. At night, the conscious mind goes to sleep, but you still have not processed some things very well. From the perspective of Chinese psychology you are "overeating": your life has things which you are trying to "eat" but cannot "swallow." For example, you may have a big project at work. You are trying to bite something and trying to chew it. TMJ is like an emotional chewing on the level of the subconscious. In the West you have the expression "Something's eating you." You are trying to chew something that you cannot chew. In some way, in the daytime you didn't finish processing the issue, so during the night, during sleep, you still continue to chew it. You also have the expression "You've bitten off more than you can chew." Very often, this health problem is related to a large amount of stress in life, like a big project or an overwhelming problem; many things are behind TMJ.

People suffering from TMJ can help themselves by massaging three special points: a point located where the bones of the thumb and index finger meet (in the web); a point located in the lower portion of the jaw muscle (the area that expands when you bite your upper and lower teeth together); and a point located in front of the ear (in the spot where there is a "hole" when the jaw is opened). Massaging these points can bring temporary relief from the side effects of TMJ, such as headaches, jaw tension and neck pain.

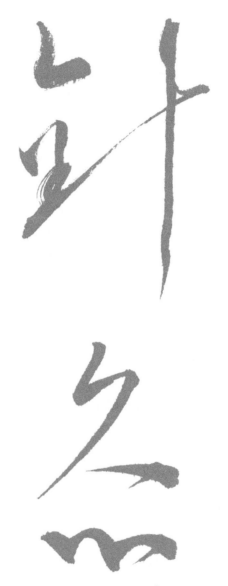

Acupuncture

If you really want to fix this kind of problem you have to learn how to let things go; you have to go to the emotions and release them. You have to understand why you are holding something beyond what you can handle. You have to understand the stress. By understanding the root cause, it will help you to release the problem. If you can learn how to let things go in an emotional way, then acupuncture and herbs will help your TMJ. Otherwise, these treatments can only provide temporary relief—a couple of months later you'll be getting it again.

Varicose Veins

I took The Dragon's Way® program and got great benefits all over. Now I'm taking it for the second time. How I can diminish the appearance and the heavy feeling caused by varicose veins?

Dr. Lu: Congratulations, you are now just beginning the real part of your healing journey. So you need to be patient and continue to practice Qigong—practice, practice, practice. As you have learned already, The Dragon's Way is designed to heal your organs and make them function well. It also makes them work better together as a whole; they rebalance and relearn how to communicate more efficiently. This will save your body a lot of Qi in the long run.

For most people, this kind of deep healing cannot be done in a short period of time. How long did you live in a certain way—with your own eating patterns and lifestyle habits—before you started on this new healing path? Deep within, your body knows how to heal itself; you were born with this program. For a few months you have been giving your body what it needs to recharge. That's why you got benefits. You need patience and dedication now to really move forward and go to the next level. Don't doubt your body's ability to clean itself

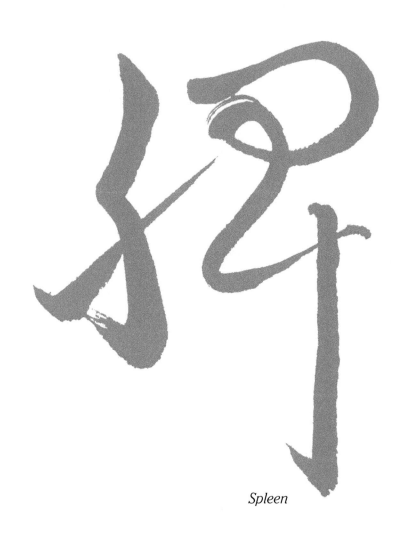

Spleen

up at the energy level and for your Qi to build and get stronger.

In The Dragon's Way there is a focus on the digestive organs: the Spleen and Stomach. You most likely remember that these two organs are very important because they are your body's main source of energy after you are born—the other is inherited Qi from your parents.

The Spleen's job is to transport food essence in the body. It also moves liquids, including blood, through your body. The Spleen controls blood flow into the many body structures it nourishes. This includes controlling how the blood flows, where it flows and how much it flows. (The Liver also has a function related to blood, but it's different than the Spleen's: the Liver stores the blood and makes sure it flows freely in your body.) Whenever there is a problem with Spleen function there will be some kind of internal bleeding. It may relate to a woman's cycle, with symptoms like heavy bleeding, an unusually long cycle, or spotting.

Another important function of the Spleen is to maintain the tone and elasticity of the blood vessel walls. If your Spleen Qi is too weak to perform this job, the blood vessel walls can become more fragile or even collapse. When this happens, the body can show several kinds of symptoms: bruising easily, chronic bleeding, and the symptom you have—varicose veins. Also, remember that dampness is the type of climatic condition related to the Spleen. If your body has internal dampness, it can create a heavy sensation.

To fix these kinds of issues you have to fix the source of the problem—weak Spleen Qi. The Spleen needs to gain more energy and to do this you have to improve its function and save as much energy as you can. You have to go deep to heal many things at the level of the root cause. If you've had the problem for a long time, it will take some time to heal. Remember, TCM is not about quick fixes; this approach treats the source and not just the symptoms.

So, please, trust your body. It loves you unconditionally and has a wisdom and timing that goes beyond what your mind can understand. Try to be peaceful during this process. From The Dragon's Way you know the Spleen is impacted by worry, anxiety and too much thinking; they can deplete the Spleen's energy. Continue with your eating for healing plan and be sure to practice Qigong. I'll say it one more time: practice, practice, practice. Qigong is what makes this program really work; the food is secondary.

Winter Blues

I'm starting to feel depressed now that winter and the holidays are here. I don't like being so busy with all the stuff you have to do at this time of year. I'm already busy enough in my life. I end up feeling tired and want to sleep through it. What advice can you give me?

Dr. Lu: Your body feels one way, but you are listening to your mind. Look at nature right now: You don't see a lot of activity, do you? The trees are not growing leaves; the flowers are not blooming! Why? What is happening? Everything is taking a good rest over the winter. There is a positive reason for everything. Nature has to rest in order to have enough energy to grow up in springtime. This is a natural cycle and everything in nature follows that Universal pattern; only humans try to go against it.

In the winter there is less light so it's natural to go to bed earlier and get up a little later. The problem for most people is their lives are not so flexible to allow this. You can choose to go more with what your body is telling you and change things so you have a little more time to relax and rest. Take some time to meditate and feel peaceful. Don't get caught in your mind and in what you think the outside world is telling you to do. You don't "have" to do anything but follow your body's wisdom and what your heart and spirit tell you. Remember, life is for the fulfillment of your enjoyment.

How to Choose a TCM Practitioner

I just moved to a different state and now I'm looking for a new TCM practitioner. Can you give me any tips to help me find someone who is really good?

Dr. Lu: First of all, I would say rely on your intuition. When you meet a practitioner, ask yourself how you really feel about this person. Don't go by reputation, fame or even a referral. You are an important and equal member in the healing partnership; you must feel that you can form a trusting bond with this person. Do you feel comfortable with him or her? Can you open up about yourself, your health and life issues? What does your "gut" really tell you?

One question to ask is this: Is your TCM practitioner really there? Is this person passionate about this work? Authentic, high-quality TCM treatment requires that practitioners be present in a unique way. They must listen carefully and actively ask questions about the symptoms you are experiencing as well as questions about your lifestyle. TCM treatment takes skill, patience and dedication. The practitioner must be able to care about you as an individual and want to work together to help you understand and resolve your health issues.

Also, be sure the practitioner is willing to spend enough time. The true essence of authentic TCM treatments is Qi, vital energy that flows through our bodies and everything in the universe. It doesn't matter what modality is used: acupuncture, acupressure or herbs. The real challenge is whether the practitioner and patient have a true connection that can spark the patient's Qi, stimulating the patient's own

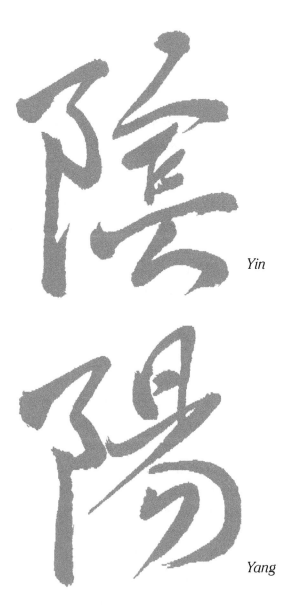

Yin

Yang

inborn capacity to heal his or her own body. Spirit is the ultimate technique. There must be an energy bond between practitioner and patient. It's the energy relationship that actually heals, not the treatment technique. Otherwise, the treatment remains superficial, staying at the physical level of symptoms and never moving deeper to reach spirit. So this work requires spending quality time, which allows the practitioner to understand underlying emotional and psychological issues, most often the root cause of health problems. You should expect to have adequate time during your appointments.

Another key point is a true TCM healer has proficient knowledge of the ancient, unchanging principles, theories and practices of traditional Chinese medicine. Good TCM doctors will use the classical four-stage diagnosis: looking, hearing and smelling, pulse-taking, and asking questions. This type of healing is serious because it deals with the energy system, a system that is even more critical to the human body than the endocrine or nervous systems. So therefore, choosing a TCM practitioner is a serious thing. A practitioner who does not have a deep understanding of the principles and practices of TCM can actually harm the patient and create more internal problems that can be very difficult to fix later on.

TCM lifestyle choices are in harmony with nature. While most people have learned from popular culture what is and isn't healthy, many would be surprised about the important differences in the TCM approach. The truth is most people know very little about the way nature works at the level of energy. A good TCM practitioner will always educate you about lifestyle choices from this point of view so that you can create a quantum difference in your healing journey. Good luck, and remember to trust your intuition.

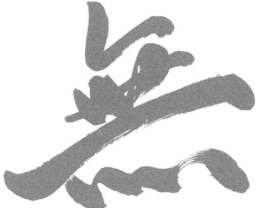

Wu

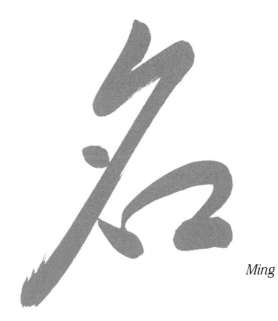

Ming

The Tao is hidden and nameless;

yet it alone knows how to render help and to fulfill.

—*Tao Te Ching,* Lao Tzu (6th century B.C.E.)

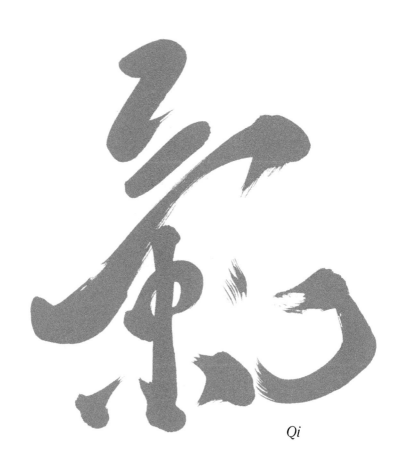

Qi

Appendix

Basic TCM Principles

TCM Principles Reflect Natural Law

The basic principles underlying the theories and practice of traditional Chinese medicine (TCM) have remained the same throughout the millennia. This is because these principles are a reflection of natural law. Ancient Chinese practitioners had a deep connection to the natural world—a quality of connection all but lost in our time. Their relationship to nature gave them a profound understanding of the intricate workings of the human body and enabled them to comprehend how it works on the invisible level of Qi, or energy.

These sages saw that following natural law—the way the universe really works—creates a foundation for health, well-being and longevity; going against nature sets the stage for illness. An example of this concept is the way we naturally feel in winter. We are almost compelled to go to bed earlier, and yet it's harder to get out of bed in the morning; the dark and cold make us want to stay indoors and hibernate. Deep within, our bodies are expressing a fundamental principle of winter: conservation and storage.

TCM principles have run as a steady current supporting the practice of authentic TCM throughout the ages. Also, TCM theories and practices have not been overturned, nor have they become outdated, precisely because they are founded on unchangeable natural law.

The Body Is an Organic Whole

Every structure in our body—tissue, bone, bowel and viscera—is an integral part of the whole. Along with the mind, emotions (which are considered actions of the mind) and spirit, they form a miraculously complex, interrelated system that is powered by energy. This is why TCM practitioners do not separate the human being into parts, nor do they treat just one part of the body.

For instance, TCM theory views the emotions as a factor related to health. It's normal to experience a range of emotions in the course of everyday life. However, when an emotion is held chronically over a period of time, it can affect the health of the whole person by disturbing the function of its associated organ. Anger, for example, impacts the function of the Liver. Yet the reverse can also be true: a Liver that is physically impaired can cause an excess of emotion, particularly anger (the emotion associated with this organ) and a stressed-out feeling.

The Body Is Inseparably Linked to Nature and the Greater Universe

Whether we are aware of it or not, the movements and changes in nature—from the cycle of the seasons to the orbit of the planets—are reflected in our bodies. Nature affects us and also, we have an impact on it.

One chapter in the *Neijing* (*The Yellow Emperor's Classic of Internal Medicine*), a TCM classic text thought to be written between 475 and 221 B.C.E., discusses the effects of altitude on health: "People who live in high areas have a long life, while those who live in low ones die young." It's interesting that modern researchers have demonstrated that mountainous areas between 5,000 and 6,500 feet above sea level are especially health-enhancing areas to live in because of the concentration of hydrogen anions. Modern issues of the human impact on weather and the environment have become very clear in recent years.

A good TCM doctor always takes into account the season, geographical location, time of day, as well as age, genetics and the condition of the individual's body in diagnosing and treating health problems. And a key TCM goal is to balance and harmonize the individual's body and being, and then harmonize that individual with nature and the universe.

Everyone Is Born with a Self-Healing Ability

TCM views the human body as a microcosm that reflects the macrocosm. Nature has a regenerative capacity, so do we. Although this ability may appear to be dormant or difficult to access in some people, especially with illness or age, it is never completely lost. It is important to know that everything you need to heal yourself exists within your being. Because it is an integrated whole, the body has all it needs to heal itself: from physical structures and processes to the energy which powers the body and enables communication right down to the most minute cellular level throughout the entire body. Helping the individual to restore this innate self-healing function is an important part of TCM treatment.

Prevention Really Is the Best Cure

Ancient Chinese doctors were paid only if their patients remained well, and prevention remains the cornerstone of TCM's approach to health. It is not unusual for TCM doctors to prescribe lifestyle changes, from diet to Qigong (a Chinese self-healing energy practice) to help restore balance. Our bodies are constantly revealing signs about the state of our health. Here in the West, it is common to ignore symptoms. In most cases they are not even viewed as signs of something gone wrong until a larger, more serious health problem has showed up. For example, broken, brittle nails seem innocuous enough, but they hint at a Liver function that is unbalanced (the nails reflect the state of the Liver's energy, according to TCM theory). For women, this symptom combined with PMS and menstrual irregularities over a period of time could indicate the potential for significant health difficulties later on. The Liver is responsible for promoting the free flow of energy and blood throughout the body, and stagnant Liver Qi is viewed by TCM as a root cause in the formation of masses and tumors.

TCM Glossary

Acupuncture

Just how long acupuncture has been practiced no one can really say. Ancient bone and stone "needles," thought to be thousands of years old, have been found in excavation sites in China. What is known is that therapy with the technique of acupuncture has been helping people heal for ages.

It's impossible to define acupuncture without linking it to the concept of Qi, or life energy. Everything in the universe is comprised of energy. In the body, Qi flows through invisible energy pathways called "meridians." Qi activates, warms and nourishes the body. Acupuncture needles—today, made of sterile stainless steel—are used to relieve energy blockages at key points (called "acupoints") along the meridians to help Qi flow smoothly. An organ's function can also be readjusted by acupuncture to restore balance to that organ as well as harmony between the organs.

Sometimes you hear people say that acupuncture hasn't worked for them. The truth of the matter is some conditions respond well to acupuncture and some don't. Also, effective treatment is dependent to a great degree on the practitioner's skill and whether his or her energy can match that of the person seeking treatment. Pain, for instance, can come from an external cause, such as a sports injury, or from an internal condition, such as a Qi deficiency or stagnation of Qi, which can show up in symptoms like a migraine headache or back pain. Generally speaking, external conditions are easier to treat. Internal conditions tend to be more complex and require a deeper knowledge to determine their root cause in order to fully resolve the health issue.

Is the key factor in acupuncture the needle, the acupoint, or the level of the practitioner? Authentic acupuncture requires deep insight into what has caused the health problem and exactly which organs have been affected. The needle is simply a vehicle between the practitioner's Qi and the patient's Qi. Bottom line, it is the understanding, skill and energy level of the acupuncturist that makes acupuncture work, and not the needles or the selection of certain acupoints.

The Five Element Theory

Supporting the body-mind-spirit understanding of human health, TCM's ancient Five Element Theory is an incredibly detailed master "blueprint" that categorizes all natural phenomena into five essential patterns or "elements." Each element—Wood, Fire, Earth, Metal and Water—is related to a season, a climate type, a pair of internal organs, an area of the body, an emotion, an aspect of the soul, sound, taste, color . . . the associations are nearly limitless. The Five Elements fundamentally set out a diagram of how nature interacts with the body and how the different dimensions of being impact each other and relate to the greater universe. This comprehensive and very powerful theory is an essential aspect of Chinese culture. The *I Ching* (*The Book of Changes*, a classic Chinese text) and disciplines such as feng shui and the Chinese martial arts have the Five Element Theory at their foundation. The profound wisdom and knowledge embedded within this theory can be applied to virtually all situations. Skilled TCM practitioners, who know how, apply it to understand the true source of health issues and effectively treat them.

Meridians

Picture a roadmap: a profusion of points woven into a web by lines of travel. Now imagine this system three-dimensionally in your body: a vast network of invisible energy pathways connecting to each other and to every atom, cell, bone, tendon, tissue, organ, each centimeter of skin—everything in your body. They link the upper portion with the lower and the surface with the interior, so that nothing is truly separate. These amazing pathways are the meridians, and they form your body into an intercommunicating whole.

Records in China as early as 722 B.C.E. describe the meridians, and the *Neijing*, a Chinese medical classic dating between 475 and 221 B.C.E., clearly states how they work: "The function of the meridian is to transport Qi and blood and circulate Yin and Yang to nourish the body." This ancient text also describes the meridians in terms of the process of disease development:

> The twelve meridians control human life,
> yet they are the place where disease can live.
> If disease starts in the meridians,
> the physician can use the meridians
> to treat the root cause of disease. —*Neijing*

There are twelve major meridians that run on each side of the body, one side mirroring the other. Each meridian corresponds to a different internal organ, and each organ, with its own unique physiological and energy functions, is not only dependent on the other organ systems but also on the greater meridian network.

Energy and blood flow continuously through the action of the meridians, yet they also transmit information to and among your organs. What kind of information? Faster than the speed of light they send signals to raise or lower your body temperature, signs that your body needs to release water, signals to regulate emotion, and so forth. Your body is constantly communicating with itself through innumerable amounts of messages passing through the meridians. They help coordinate the work of the organs and keep your body balanced by regulating its energy functions.

According to TCM theory, as long as sufficient Qi flows freely through the meridians and your organs work in harmony your body can remain healthy. This means that when your body's meridian system functions well, you are well. Yet just like roadways to a city, they can become clogged or blocked. When this happens it affects the function of the corresponding organ and ultimately the whole body.

The beauty of meridians is their great sensitivity—they can carry the effects of stimulation in the form of healing energy throughout your entire body. It is this quality that allows the various forms of TCM treatment to work: acupuncture, acupressure, Chinese herbs, foods, Five Element psychology, and Qigong. Through the use of these modalities, the flow of energy in the meridians can be affected, restoring the balance and health of the individual.

Qi

Qi is the life force that permeates everything in the universe. Without it there can be no growth and change. Your physical body cannot exist without Qi. When you die your Qi leaves—it's transformed.

It's true that Qi is "energy," as it's usually translated, but this aspect of Qi relating to power or animating force is just one side of the whole picture. The other side of Qi is intelligence and function. What does this mean exactly? Have you ever wondered how the rising and ebbing tide keeps perfect pace with the lunar cycle? How a tree knows it's time to sprout leaves? How your body feels the season has changed from winter to spring and adjusts its own internal rhythms? It is Qi that allows all things to communicate with each other at an invisible level. Qi carries infinite messages and pieces of information, connecting all dimensions.

In your body this invisible life force travels in pathways, called "meridians," that form an intricate network, connecting all areas and systems. Each of your organs has a different type of Qi, a unique message, a certain "frequency" related to its specific function. Think of a TV. The electricity is the energy/power aspect of Qi, and the intelligence aspect is the proper function of the internal components (in your body, your organs) that allows the set to receive the frequencies of the various channels. Both aspects are needed to have a functioning whole: the power of Qi needs the intelligence of Qi to give it direction and refinement of function.

Qigong

At the very center of Qigong is Qi, the vital life energy that animates everything in the universe, including the body. Although it is a practice that uses movements and postures and can create many physical healing benefits, Qigong is *not* physical exercise. It moves beyond the physical level of muscle and tissue and works at the level of Qi. Literally meaning "energy work," Qigong breaks down energy blockages and promotes the free flow of energy throughout your body's meridian system, the invisible pathways through which Qi moves and that connect everything in your body. Consistent Qigong practice increases and balances your body's Qi. Working directly on the meridian system—your energy body—it stimulates and nourishes the internal organs, making the energetic communication between them more efficient. And by increasing the effectiveness of all body systems, Qigong helps conserve Qi. These qualities are important to health because TCM theory holds that in order to have good health you must have sufficient Qi and your internal organs must function together in harmony.

This ancient self-healing practice can also convey many spiritual benefits. Qigong has the ability to enhance sensitivity, develop intuition and expand your perception, especially how you view the world, life, and *your* life, in particular. It integrates the body, mind and spirit, promoting physical health, peace of mind and harmony of spirit. Further, it creates harmony of the self with the Universal—viewed as the deepest source of healing in the Chinese tradition. In essence, Qigong moves you far beyond the five senses, allowing you to tap into the healing energy of the universe.

Tao

Tao is the one thing that cannot be defined. "Tao defined is not the constant Tao. No name names its eternal name." So states the very opening chapter of the *Tao Te Ching*, the classic Taoist text ascribed to the great master Lao Tzu, who lived in sixth century B.C.E. China.

Right from the start, this ancient sage warns us about words and language. A word stands for the thing it represents, yet a word is an abstraction—it can never contain or convey the experience or essence of that very thing. The word "flower" is instantly understood by most, yet everyone might have a completely different flower in mind—a yellow daffodil for one person, a dark purple orchid for another. And no matter what appears on our mental screen, it simply cannot give anything of the sensation of that flower against your skin or its aroma wafting through the air—or the feeling in your heart when someone gives you a flower.

One thing seems clear: If you remain at the level of words, you stay in the mind; if you move into the senses, you come to know the body; if you fall into your Heart you arrive at the gateway to Tao, for the Heart is the dwelling place of our spirit, which connects us with the deepest experience of all that is and all that is unseen. The Chinese character for "Tao" means "the Way" or "the Path." It is Nature, the way of Nature. Following Tao is to flow with that force, both in terms of attuning ourselves with the Universal, the external natural world around us, and following—being true to—our own inner nature. When these three alignments intersect, we create the ground for oneness with the eternal Tao.

Yin and Yang

"If you can understand Yin and Yang you can hold the universe in your hands," says a classical Chinese text. This is the power and pervasiveness ancient TCM texts invested in these two universal energies.

Everything is composed of Yin and Yang. A part of natural law, they are two opposite yet complementary energies, never separate, always interdependent. This interpenetrating, inseparable relationship is reflected in the circular Yin-Yang symbol. The small dots within each of the two energies symbolize that there is always some Yin within Yang and vice versa. Nothing is absolute—the designation of something as

Yin or Yang is always relative to some other thing. For example, day is considered Yang, yet within every day is a Yang part, the early morning, and a Yin part, late day as it begins to turn to night. There is a dynamic dance between Yin and Yang: they constantly turn from one to the other and back again. Nothing about them is static. In the natural world this phenomenon is seen in the changing of the seasons: the cold of winter yields to the warmth of spring and summer heat, and then gradually turns cool in fall to become winter once again. The theory of Yin and Yang is fundamental to the practice of TCM in terms of understanding, diagnosing and treating health difficulties.

TCM and Food

TCM Wisdom on What to Eat

TCM advises following the seasons when selecting which foods to eat. This means choosing foods that are available naturally in season as well as keeping in mind and balancing the specific taste or flavor associated with each season. Each of the Five Elements has an associated flavor:

Fire (Heart) – Bitter
Earth (Spleen) – Sweet
Metal (Lung) – Spicy
Water (Kidney) – Salty
Wood (Liver) – Sour

There are many helpful tips, some taken from thousands of years of TCM wisdom, regarding eating.

Try to use your intuition when selecting foods at the market. Go with the first idea that comes into your mind. Generally that is what your body needs. There is a learning curve to this; it takes practice and patience.

Eat cooked and not raw foods. Raw foods have a cold essence, and the Stomach, according to TCM, has a "preference" for warm food. Foods with a cold essence unbalance the Stomach. Cold foods in terms of temperature also impair the function of the Stomach and inhibit the digestive process. Avoid cold drinks and beverages for the same reason.

Eat fried and spicy foods and drink alcohol in moderation. These foods and drinks create internal heat in the body. Meat also is a burden on the digestive system, so try to limit it in your diet.

Don't choose nonfat and decaffeinated products. The chemicals used in the production of these items are worse for you than the fat or caffeine in the unadulterated products.

TCM Wisdom on How to Eat

TCM understands that the way in which you eat is almost as important as what you eat. The following tips will help you maximize the value of the food in your daily diet.

Eat the greatest quantity of food earlier in the day. While you are up and active, your body needs a good foundation of nutrition. Also, eat heavier foods earlier in the day so that they can be thoroughly digested.

Eat at regular intervals during the day. The Stomach and Spleen need an adequate supply of food to digest and refine steadily throughout the day in order to make an important daily energy resource for your body.

Try not to overeat at each meal. Ideally, you should stop when you are about seventy percent full. This way, the digestive organs will not be taxed by trying to process too much food at one time. An overloaded stomach places an energy drain on the entire body. Overeating can result in retention of undigested food and indigestion, causing symptoms such as abdominal distension, gas and vomiting.

Avoid eating late at night or just before bedtime. These habits force your digestive organs to work overtime digesting food when they naturally should be resting and restoring themselves while you sleep.

Eat "softly." Try to maintain a quiet, relaxed manner while eating. Refrain from too much conversation during meals. Talking and eating at the same time reverses the energy relationship between the Lung and the Stomach.

Eat in an unhurried way. Don't eat while working or rush away from the table directly back to work or another activity.

Chew your food thoroughly. This practice makes the digestive process much easier for the body as a whole.

Resources

Nan Lu, OMD

Nan Lu, OMD, is a classically and academically trained doctor of traditional Chinese medicine in private practice in New York City. A Taoist Qigong master and internationally recognized Taiji champion, Dr. Lu is also an author and educator and the creator of numerous Taoist-based healing programs. He founded Traditional Chinese Medicine World Foundation in 1995 and continues to serve as its director. Guiding this not-for-profit organization, Dr. Lu creates and oversees ongoing initiatives that encompass professional curricula as well as self-healing programs and resources to help individuals achieve optimum health through TCM. Dr. Lu is the author of numerous articles, columns and a blog, *AskDrLu.com*. He has also authored three best-selling self-care books on traditional Chinese medicine, originally published by HarperCollins. A clinical associate professor at the School for Social Welfare, State University of New York (SUNY) at Stony Brook, Dr. Lu serves as an executive board member of its Center for Culturally Competent Education and Training.

Tao of Healing Center

Nan Lu, OMD, maintains a private practice in New York City at Tao of Healing Center. In additional to individual sessions, Tao of Healing also holds classes, workshops and intensive training to further self-cultivation of energy, health and spiritual growth.

With a goal to help individuals awaken the healing power they were born with, the Center offers Taoist healing programs, which are taught under Dr. Lu's direction or by his students who have received his permission to teach. Tao of Healing is dedicated to serving as the source for authentic information and training in Taoist internal martial arts and Taoist healing knowledge.

Tao of Healing programs help participants achieve optimal health and cultivate spiritual growth to unlock each individual's unique wisdom and power. The heart of this healing approach stems from *Wu Ming* Qigong, an internal martial arts system descended directly from the ancient Taoist masters Lao Tzu and Chuang Tzu. Tao of Healing programs include beginner and advanced *Wu Ming* Qigong, Taiji: Beyond the Martial Arts, Taiji Sword, and Life Force: Tao of Medical Qigong, an intensive training for those who want to become an energy practitioner.

For information on Tao of Healing and its programs please visit www.taoofhealing.com.

Traditional Chinese Medicine World Foundation

Founded in 1995 by Nan Lu, OMD, Traditional Chinese Medicine World Foundation is a not-for-profit organization based in New York City. The Foundation is committed to building bridges of understanding between East and West through educational programs based on traditional Chinese medicine (TCM), Taoist healing and classical Chinese martial arts. Its goal is to advance the understanding and implementation of authentic TCM.

One of the oldest, continually practiced medical systems in the world, TCM is based on natural law with the aim of restoring balance and harmony at the body-mind-spirit level, which reawakens and enhances an individual's self-healing ability. The TCM paradigm has major implications for how we heal from disease, how we stay healthy, how we relate to ourselves, others and our environment, and how we expand our healing potential. In addition to offering educational programs, Traditional Chinese Medicine World Foundation serves as an information resource and develops creative outreach initiatives on authentic TCM, Taoist healing and the classical Chinese martial arts.

The Foundation's educational efforts focus on TCM philosophy, theories and modalities, which include acupuncture, acupressure, classical Chinese herbal therapy, internal martial arts like Qigong and Taiji, the prescription of food for healing, and Five Element psychology—an ancient Chinese form of working with the mind and emotions based on TCM's Five Element Theory. The Foundation's educational outreach is geared toward the general public and medical and healthcare professionals, as well as organizations from both mainstream and complementary and alternative medicine (CAM) communities.

Traditional Chinese Medicine World Foundation seeks to broaden the potential for healing and improved quality of life for the individual and society. Foundation programming and learning resources provide authentic information and experiential learning about TCM and its understanding of vital energy (Qi), the body's natural ability to heal itself, and the essential role of belief systems and consciousness in healing. The Foundation believes TCM offers the promise of filling gaps in current medical care, especially for chronic, intractable conditions such as cancer, pain and immune disorders. Complementary use of TCM with Western medicine can have a synergistic effect, making treatments more effective when used together.

The Foundation hosts three websites: www.tcmworld.org, www.tcmconference.org and www.breastcancer.com.

Programs of Traditional Chinese Medicine World Foundation

The following programs were created by Nan Lu, OMD, and are offered by Traditional Chinese Medicine World Foundation.

Breast Cancer Prevention Project (BCPP)

True prevention for breast health is an active, life-enhancing process. From the TCM perspective, it can only be achieved by developing and maintaining a strong energy system. Life force or the intelligent energy that powers the body's organ systems must flow smoothly throughout the body and the organ systems have to work in harmony. The Breast Cancer Prevention Project (BCPP) is an educational initiative that communicates this sound TCM healing wisdom. It also offers *Wu Ming* Qigong for Breast Health, a unique training program that teaches breast health energy movements to individuals and healthcare professionals so they can share the TCM approach to prevention with others.

Please visit www.breastcancer.com and www.tcmworld.org for information and resources.

The Dragon's Way® Weight Loss and Stress Management Program

The Dragon's Way is a ground-breaking wellness program based on TCM principles. Through simple Qigong energy movements and an eating for healing plan, it allows the body to rebalance and renew itself, reconnecting with its innate self-healing ability. The Dragon's Way is unique among weight loss approaches because it works on the invisible level of energy, building Qi deep within the body. Participants learn how a host of common conditions, including excess weight, high blood pressure, high cholesterol, anxiety and various forms of chronic pain, are the body's way of signaling that it is out of balance. The program helps participants learn to identify and listen to these important messages and address the root cause of body imbalances. It teaches time-tested TCM tools and strategies for creating a healthy body and a happy life through balance and harmony with nature. Certified

Dragon's Way instructors guide program participants through an informative, educational and enjoyable six-week program that changes life perspectives and lives.

For program information and locations, visit www.tcmworld.org.

The Dragon's Way® Weight Loss and Stress Management Program – Certified Instructor Training

For healthcare practitioners or anyone who has a passion to work with individuals, helping them learn how to connect to their true healing potential, The Dragon's Way Certified Instructor Training Program offers a special opportunity. With a strong focus on Qigong practice, The Dragon's Way Weight Loss and Stress Management Program has helped thousands of individuals rebalance their bodies, build a strong energy foundation, let go of health conditions and achieve a state of wellness they never thought possible. The Certified Instructor Training Program is an immersion experience in the self-healing powers of Qigong and TCM. Instructor trainees focus on the cultivation of their own personal energy, or Qi, and receive in-depth instruction on how to teach the popular six-week Dragon's Way Program. Trainees learn about the principles and theories of TCM, the energy essence of special healing foods, and how to teach The Dragon's Way Qigong movements. Once certified, instructors can share this powerful healing knowledge with their family, friends and community.

To learn more about this unique instructor training opportunity, please visit www.tcmworld.org.

Finding Freedom Retreats

Finding Freedom is a weekend retreat that helps participants rediscover their own self-healing ability and reconnect to the freedom of their spirit. Offered several times throughout the year in varying locations around the country, Finding Freedom creates a peaceful, nurturing and enjoyable space that allows for a deeper kind of healing. It's a special retreat where participants learn how to apply the knowledge and wisdom of TCM to uplift and change their lives. *Wu Ming* Qigong practice helps build internal energy and rebalance the body-mind-spirit, fostering harmony and a sense of well-being.

Please visit www.tcmworld.org for information about Finding Freedom retreats.

Conference: Building Bridges of Integration for Traditional Chinese Medicine

Truly a profound learning experience in a healing environment, this unique TCM conference, held since 2002, is vibrant, engaging and fun. Dynamic and inspiring presenters share their insight and perspectives on TCM and authentic body-mind-spirit healing. Individuals and professionals from a diverse range of healthcare practices gather with the purpose of stepping into an unusual world of energy. There, they discover how to nurture the body, mind and spirit and learn new ways to expand their own understanding and growth as well as help others.

For information on Building Bridges for TCM conferences visit www.tcmconference.org and www.tcmworld.org.

CPSIA information can be obtained
at www.ICGtesting.com
Printed in the USA
BVHW080153240119
538466BV00007BA/490/P